THE NAUTILUS® HOME FITNESS WORKOUT BOOK

THE NAUTILUS® HOME FITNESS WORKOUT BOOK

MICHAEL D. WOLF, Ph.D.

CONTEMPORARY
BOOKS, INC.
CHICAGO

The term "Nautilus" is a registered trademark of Nautilus Sports/Medical Industries, Inc. There is no affiliation between Nautilus Sports/Medical Industries and the author or publisher of this book. Neither this book nor its contents are sponsored, authorized, or approved by nautilus Sports/Medical Industries.

Published by Contemporary Books, Inc.
180 North Michigan Avenue, Chicago, Illinois 60601
Manufactured in the United States of America
International Standard Book Number: 0-8092-5260-0

Published simultaneously in Canada by Beaverbooks, Ltd.
195 Allstate Parkway, Valleywood Business Park
Markham, Ontario L3R 4T8 Canada

CONTENTS

ACKNOWLEDGMENTS

My sincere thanks to those who made it all happen:

My wife Marti Ann, ace photographer of the exercise world, who shot her first cover, her fifth set of interior photos, and did the photo-styling as well;

Editor-in-Chief Nancy Crossman, who stroked and tanned on a Florida golf course while I slaved at the word processor;

All-around star Boushelle Peabody Alvarez, who graced the interior pages as our Abdominal Machine model and did double duty as our makeup and hair stylist;

Michael Petty, the man on the Back Machine (inside and out), who by day gets New York City fit;

Cover girl Anna Lee, a top pro model who fortunately happens to be the girl next door;

Marti Ann's great photo assistant, Bart Everly;

John Grande of the John Grande Photo Studio, for his space and his help;

Steve Kass, Bruce Frankel, and Howard Saunders of American Leisure Facilities Management Corp., who kindly housed our machines during their New York visit; and

Marty Shapiro (Keeper of the Kaypro) and Zoilo Ruiz (who could have gotten it for me cheaper), for being true friends.

THE NAUTILUS® HOME FITNESS WORKOUT BOOK

1

INTRODUCTION

More than you know, you've just taken a major step toward health, fitness, and enhanced physical and mental performance. You may have bought the New Nautilus Home Abdominal Machine just to trim that slightly rounded midsection or the Back Machine to fight off the back trouble that plagues so many American adults. Good move! For the first time, you can perform graded intensity exercise—at home—for your back and abdomen. No more endless repetitions of sit-ups and back extensions. With ten levels of intensity, you can continually challenge your body as it grows stronger.

But there's more! You're also about to give yourself a powerful new foundation for movement. The abdominal and lower back muscles form the very core of effective physical performance. Coordinated and powerful movements of the arms and legs always start from the power base of a fit torso. But you don't have to be a professional athlete, or even a weekend athlete, to feel the boost. Plain and simple, if you move, you'll see the difference that a fit middle makes! Of course, if you *do* hit a ball around once in a while, or swim, or run, you'll be very pleasantly surprised at the new power your torso adds to the movement.

THE BATTLE PLAN

There's more to a trim middle and a strong, healthy back than you were led to believe by the ads, though. You can't just jump on your new Nautilus machines, work away, and reap the benefits in no time flat. The instruction manual that came with your machine(s) painted far too simple a picture. To do it right—meaning *safely* and *most effectively*—you'll need to read this book and follow the plan. If you're *really* after a healthy back and a flat midsection, you've no choice. Total home abdominal and back fitness demands all of the following:

- a proper warm-up and stretch
- correct use of the machines
- an additional exercise or two to attack the tough-to-reach muscles of the abdomen and back
- a combination of proper diet and aerobic exercise

Why so complicated? Here's a point-by-point explanation.

Proper warm-up and stretch. As noted above, you can now, for the first time, perform progressively loaded exercise for your stomach and back at home. You're no longer performing those lower-intensity sit-ups or back extensions, which don't require much preparation. You're now going to be challenging your body as never before, and you are *at risk* if you don't realize it and get ready for it! I probably don't have to tell you that those aren't toys you've purchased. Especially before using the Back Machine, you'll need to stretch and do a warm-up set of repetitions (more on this in Chapter 4).

Correct use of the machines. This one *almost* speaks for itself. The most powerful tool can be rendered useless or even dangerous if used incorrectly. For example, one of my discoveries in test-driving the machines was that the level 2 setting on both units is set by putting the pin in the *first* hole.

Example number two is the existence of a two-position intensity option on the Back Machine. What's that you ask? The Back Machine comes to you with the lever arms set at the *more* difficult of the two settings. I was surprised by the difficulty of the "easy" levels on the machine. (I can pretty handily work at 100 pounds on the commercial version of the Back Machine.) You'll need to find the necessary tools—a screwdriver and vise-grip pliers—and switch to the easier setting (see photo on page 24). You'll notice a major difference. I advise *all* of you to make the switch.

The need for ancillary exercises. If you did nothing more with your back or abdominal muscles than bend forward or backward, and if you didn't possess muscles that crisscross the abdomen (giving you the potential for a super-effective natural girdle), there would be no need for exercises to supplement your Nautilus work. But since you *do* bend and twist in an infinite number of ways, and since the internal and external obliques and transverse abdominus (page 14) are waiting for you to whip them into shape, you're going to supplement your three-times-a-week Nautilus work with the special program that's laid out in Chapter 5. And for those of you who purchased just one of the two machines, these special ancillary exercises will go far toward taking the other's place.

The need for aerobic exercise and nutritional smarts. Forget the thinly veiled implications in those Nautilus ads that three-times-a-week use of the Abdominal Machine will burn body fat right off your stomach. It just isn't so. Real, hard research, supervised by Dr. Frank I. Katch, chairman of the Department of Exercise Science at the University of Massachusetts (Amherst), has just conclusively shown that *you cannot spot reduce*.

Though my colleagues and I have absolutely struggled to convince the American public of this, many of you still are under the impression that sit-ups will burn fat off your stomach and leg lifts will burn fat off your thighs. I can't tell you how sorry I am that it's not true! The human body can use stored fat for energy by drawing it from programmed-in sites. You do not and cannot choose these locations. Exercising the muscles of the abdomen will not necessarily lead to a reduction of body fat in that area. If your body is genetically programmed to break down fat stored in the thighs first, that's where it will come from, no matter which muscles you're exercising.

Even *more* important, fat is only a minor source of energy for exercise that lasts five minutes or less. Your Nautilus Home Abdominal Machine has no match in what it can do for the muscles in that region, but you *will not* burn the body fat that lies above those muscles without some carefully structured aerobic exercise and some attention to what and how you eat. (Aerobic exercise, discussed in Chapter 6, is the true key to the control of body fat.)

THE BOTTOM LINE

Take the time to read through the book and digest what I'm offering. I'm not telling you all this because I'm some zealous believer in ridiculously hard work and dietary sacrifice. It's *your* best interests I have at heart! In your hands is the key to a trimmer and healthier torso than you ever dreamed possible, and the program is safe, besides being effective. Give it your best shot!

2 THE NAUTILUS MYSTIQUE

If some visitor from another planet were to observe the record-breaking sales of machines that train just one muscle group, they'd have to conclude that buyers had awfully high confidence in the manufacturer! How was such confidence built? What makes Nautilus so special? Sit back and listen to the tale.

A BETTER BARBELL

The man behind Nautilus Sports/Medical Industries, Inc., is Arthur A. Jones. While the ideas and prototypes percolated for perhaps 30 years or more as he globe-trotted in a series of Indiana Jones–type adventures, Jones began the actual Nautilus company in tiny Lake Helen, Florida, in 1970.

As legend tells it, the name Nautilus was coined by one of Mr. Jones's sons, who noted the similarity between the sea-dwelling Nautilus creature and his father's groundbreaking addition to strength training—the cam.

Jones knew, from a lifetime of weightlifting and a study of the human body, that barbells left much to be desired. The advent of weightlifting machines surely addressed some of the safety and convenience problems (no more weights to drop on your foot or your neck), but the major problem of strength training remained. Jones saw the fundamental difference between how human muscle and bone produced force and how barbells and machines resisted that force. And he vowed to eliminate the difference.

The situation is this: We still have a long way to go in understanding exactly how and why muscle responds to strength training. What we *do* know is that, if a muscle is forced to overcome resistance, it will grow. Furthermore, it appears that, if the resistance is structured carefully, muscle will grow bigger faster. And therein lies the rub. How do you build a better strength training mousetrap?

First, you need to understand muscle and bone. As it turns out, each and every muscle in the body performs in a peculiar way based on its own internal structure and how it attaches to bone. From a fully stretched position, some muscles appear to get stronger and stronger as they contract. That is, if you were to measure the amount of force the muscle could create, the number would get higher as the muscle went from the stretched to the fully contracted position. So far, so good.

Other muscles, though, actually create great force when in their fully elongated position but yield less and less force as they contract through their range. And then there are other muscles that create little force in the stretched position, great force in the middle range of their contraction, and little force again at the end of the range. (Many of us ask each night: "Why does it have to be so complicated?")

As if that weren't enough, barbells and weight machines follow their own laws of physics, too. Here's a true-false question to test your intellect (and whether you've read my other two Nautilus books):

T or F: A 30-pound barbell always gives the muscle 30 pounds of resistance.
Answer: False.

As a barbell is moved through space, those old laws of physics dictate how the effective resistance seen by the muscle, or the *torque*, will change. Sometimes, as in a Standing Biceps Curl, a 30-pound barbell starts with a very low *torque,* reaches its maximum difficulty at exactly the halfway point (arms parallel to the floor), then gets easier as the movement is completed. This is wonderful news, considering that, while the barbell's resistance changes in one way, the muscle may be creating force in a totally different pattern.

Case in point: your hamstrings, the group of muscles on the backs of your thighs, are at their strongest when almost fully extended. In an exercise in which you lie in a prone position and bring your heels to your buttocks by bending at the knees, the hamstrings get weaker and weaker as they contract. It just so happens that in many machines the laws of physics dictate that the weight you choose to lift actually gets *harder* as you contract. What happens then? At the exact point where the hamstrings become too weak to overcome the increasing difficulty of the weight being lifted, you fail. Exercise over. Period. And you've terminated the exercise before giving your hamstrings the amount of work required to make them grow most effectively.

Arthur Jones knew all this. What he did was create an intelligent barbell, or what he calls a "thinking man's barbell." The Nautilus cam, the invention that gave birth to the company name, actually changes the resistance that the weight stack shows to the muscle. Choosing 30 pounds (or hole number 3) on a Nautilus machine means that your muscles will be working against a resistance that varies around the 30-pound number *in direct concert* with how that particular muscle changes in its own force production ability. Each Nautilus machine has its own specially designed cam, since each muscle has a unique "strength curve." If the muscle to be trained on a particular machine starts off weak, gets stronger, then declines in force production ability, the Nautilus cam will take the 30 pounds and change it. How is this magic trick pulled off?

It's all in the cam, an off-round wheel. You should remember from those ancient math clases that a circle has a constant radius (the distance from the center of the circle to the perimeter). A cam can be described as having a changing radius. It may get larger as the cam spins, or it may get smaller, or it may vary in any desired fashion. Aha! you say. Isn't there some vague similarity between the varying ability of human muscle to create force and the varying radius of the cam? Yes. There's more than a vague similarity. It's, in fact, how Jones's Nautilus machines work their magic.

Though the actual process remains seen by few human eyes, (I was research coordinator and never got to witness it), Nautilus reportedly and apparently, since its machines work so well, designs the cam for each machine specifically to match the muscle being trained. In the case of the Nautilus Leg Curl, which trains the hamstrings, the cam makes the 30 pounds lighter and lighter as the heels approach the buttocks. While the actual variation may be only three or four pounds in either direction, the cam makes a pronounced difference.

In the case of your new home machines, a cam is visible only inside the abdominal machine. (It's got teeth and is hard to miss if you take a peek.) My deduction is that the variation in resistance required in the Back Machine can be accomplished through the simple mechanical linkage used in place of a cam.

Enough physics! What does this mean for your stomach and back? It means *time efficiency*. It means that every repetition of every set is stressing your muscles in synchrony with their biomechanical patterns. It means that you'll get better results in less time. That's my favorite deal. What's the whole thing called? *Variable resistance*.

WHAT ELSE MAKES NAUTILUS SPECIAL?

Mr. Jones designs a host of other features into his machines. Even the first units, some of which can still be found in the dark recesses of Nautilus–Lake Helen and on Jones's ranch in Ocala, show off the design ingenuity he brought to strength training. You can likewise find all of them on the new home machines. There are seven, besides the variable resistance feature offered by the cam. They are:

- resistance through the full range of motion
- direct resistance
- rotary resistance
- positive and negative work
- stretching in the starting position
- resistance in the fully contracted position
- unlimited speed of movement

Here's a brief summary for those of you who really want to know or who enjoy learning about mechanical devices.

Resistance through the full range of motion. For a muscle to be maximally stimulated to grow, it must be trained through its entire range of motion. Hold one arm outstretched in front of your torso, palm up. Bring the hand to the shoulder, bending at the elbow. That entire movement is called the *range of motion.* Training your biceps and brachialis through anything less than that range will simply not give you as fast and complete results.

Nautilus machines are well known for their ability to train muscles through the full range of motion, and the new home machines are no exception. Those of you who've already taken them for a ride know what I'm talking about.

Direct resistance. If you were to forge a chain of 10 links, with 9 being able to withstand 100 pounds of force, but the 10th capable of holding only 80, it takes no great engineering acumen to predict the result of an 81-pound tug. A chain is only as strong as its weakest link.

What does this bit of physics have to do with your body? Should you attempt to train a muscle that is a step or two removed from the weight stack or resistance—say by a smaller and weaker muscle—the weak link will break before the stronger ones. Any strength exercise involving the hand grip could be used as an example. What happens if the small and relatively weak muscles in the forearm and hand are incapable of holding a barbell or chin-up bar? You let go, frequently before the larger and more powerful muscles of the upper arm or torso have gotten the work they need to grow maximally. If the hands go, there goes the exercise.

Wouldn't it be nice if you could train the large muscles without letting the smaller ones intervene (assuming you have the time and ability to train the smaller muscles afterward)? That's what Nautilus's direct resistance principle is about. Wherever possible, the muscle to be trained *directly* applies the force against the machine, preventing the intrusion of weak links. Both of the new home machines feature this principle—the torso pressing directly against the machines' movement arms and pads.

Rotary resistance. All human movement is accomplished through the rotation of bones around joints. Frequently, the actual movement path is circular (like your hand in the earlier biceps curl example). If you combine the rotation of two joints, you may get a straight-line path. (Lift your hand straight over head. There's rotation at the elbow and shoulder.) For maximum safety, comfort, and effectiveness, the machine you're training on should let you match its axis of rotation with your own. In other words, in an Abdominal Curl or Back Extension, the point around which your torso rotates should match the point around which the machine's movement arm rotates. In the Nautilus Home Back Machine, it's built-in—no adjustments are necessary for proper rotational alignment. The axis-to-axis match in the Home Abdominal Machine is accomplished by setting correct seat height. (See Chapter 4.)

Positive and negative work. You don't want to read, and I don't want to write, a scholarly dissertation on what these creatures are. You can, however, read all about it in my book, *The Complete Book of Nautilus Training*. In brief, a muscle performs positive, or *concentric*, work when it contracts or shortens (that biceps curl example again). If a muscle attempts to contract but is pulled out or lengthened by a *greater* force, it is said to be performing a negative, or *eccentric*, contraction. Picture yourself hanging from a chin-up bar (by your hands, silly, not your neck). Once your muscles fatigue and gravity starts winning the battle, you'll start dropping. The muscles are still trying to contract, but gravity's pull is greater than the force they can create. They are in an eccentric mode.

Suffice it to say that most authorities these days, present company included, consider the negative phase of every repetition critically important to training gains. That is, it's not good enough to raise a weight carefully, or contract in a positive mode, then just drop the weight back to starting position. Maximum gains will come to those who work slowly and diligently in both the positive *and* negative phases of the contraction. (See Chapter 4 for specific instructions.)

Stretching in the starting position. Here's another trick to wring maximum results out of your training. If the muscle is stretched just beyond its normal length (not always possible, by the way), you'll see both greater training gains and a maintenance, if not actual improvement, in flexibility. The Home Back Machine does this really well. The Abdominal Machine obviously proved resistant to the concept, since you are not placed in a stretched position to start the exercise. (Sometimes the contortions that would be required to obtain this prestretch are simply not feasible or practical.) Just how much you'll suffer is open to question. It's certainly no reason to send the unit back to Virginia, however.

Resistance in the fully contracted position. Here's another one of those fancy tricks that squeezes the last little training gain out of exercise. A machine that offers resistance in the position of full contraction prevents you from resting at the end of a repetition, thereby keeping the muscles working, or *loaded,* at all times. You'll find yourself wishing Nautilus hadn't designed this feature in, but it means better results, so don't worry about it.

Unlimited speed of movement. The wiser among you have already concluded from the title of this section that machines exist that *do* limit the speed of movement. Many experts feel that a strength training device should allow you to move through the range of motion at a speed of your own choosing, with room for natural acceleration and deceleration. The research is far from conclusive, and since constant-velocity abdominal machines don't exist and the only constant-velocity back machine costs about $25,000, you should follow the advice in Chapter 4 on how fast to move on your new machine(s).

GRADUATION DAY

You're now a proud graduate of the Short Course on Nautilus. Congratulations. Your degree is worth absolutely nothing on the open market, but it may be quite useful at the next cocktail party or lunch at the health spa.

Your total torso program draws near. Read on.

3 WHAT'S WRONG WITH SIT-UPS AND BACK EXTENSIONS?

Though thousands of you have bought the new Nautilus home machines, a far greater number are unconvinced that there's anything wrong with Sit-Ups, Leg Lifts, and Back Extensions. While correctly performed calisthenics like Curl-Ups and Back Extensions do offer positive results, a scientific rationale *does* exist for the expenditure of money on dedicated machines.

FLATTEN YOUR STOMACH BUT RUIN YOUR BACK

The chances are quite high that you, like millions of other Americans, were—or, heaven forbid, still are—doing your daily Sit-Ups with your feet wedged under some environmental restraint. It was the way you and all of us were taught "way back then." Similarly, many of you are lying on your back and watching the Hollywood exercise gurus lead you in leg lifts. Unfortunately, exercise didn't become a science in this country until very recently, and the few people who understood how the body worked before that evidently didn't exercise! Those old Sit-Ups were doing more harm than good, Leg Lifts are nothing short of suicidal, and it's only in the past few years that we've come to those frightening conclusions.

How could the innocent Sit-Up, which after all uses the muscles on the front of the torso, harm the back? And Leg Lifts, the absolute mainstay of American abdominal exercise—how could *they* be doing more harm than good? The culprit was and still is a muscle group called the *iliopsoas.* Remember that word, for if you have back pain, your "psoas" may very likely be the cause.

The muscle that most obviously raises your torso in a Sit-Up is the rectus abdominus (see Figure 1 on page 14). As muscles generally do, it runs from one bone to another. When one of those bones is held steady, and the muscle contracts, the other must move. Let's perform a simple demonstration to make that point clear, using the biceps muscle on the front of your upper arm.

With this book in your hand, and keeping the elbow motionless, lift the book toward your shoulder. What you have done is to stabilize the shoulder, the area to which the biceps attach. With that region held motionless, a contraction of the biceps pulls on the forearm, the other attachment, and the hand moves.

Now for the real test. Find your way to a desk or table and sit facing it with one hand under the top. Contract your biceps in an attempt to lift the table, but let your upper torso and shoulder move freely. What happens? With the forearm now held stationary, the other biceps attachment, the shoulder, will move. The point to be made is that, when one attachment is stabilized, the other will move when the muscle contracts.

What does all this have to do with Sit-Ups, Leg Lifts, and your lower back? Just a little more anatomy and you'll see the picture clearly. The rectus abdominus runs from the pelvis to the sternum (breastbone). You now know that, if the pelvis is stabilized and the rectus contracts, the sternum will move. There's your Sit-Up, right? Hold the lower body down, contract the abdominals, and lift the torso, right? Sorry—that's only half the story. And the Leg Lift: Since the rectus abdominus doesn't attach to the legs, why does it feel like you're using it anyway? It's our old friend the psoas that complicates the picture.

Researchers in the field of biomechanics, the study of the

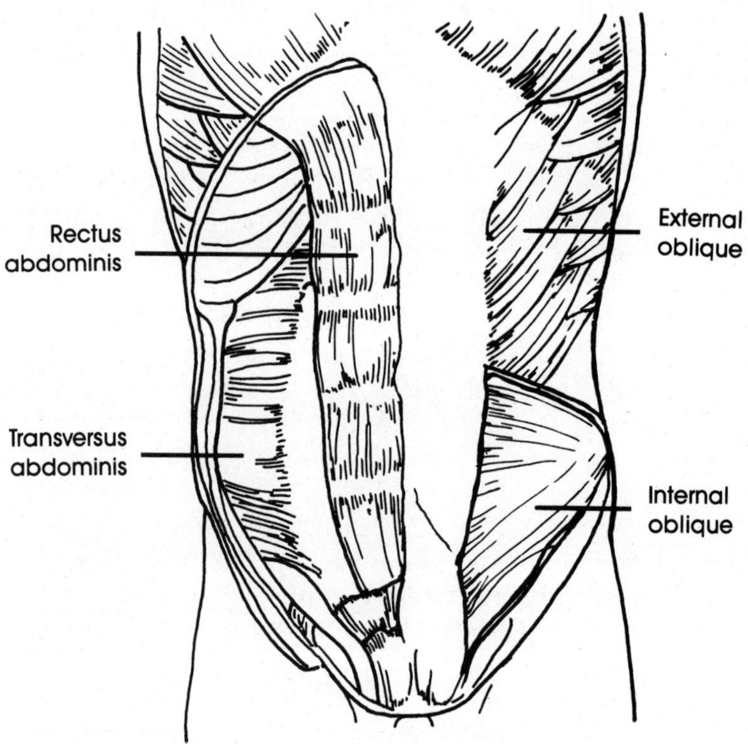

Primary muscles of the front torso.

physics of human movement, revealed that the psoas, under the right conditions (or actually, for your back, the *wrong* conditions), could do more work than the abdominals in lifting the torso in a Sit-Up and was the major muscle group responsible for holding the legs aloft in the Leg Lift. The reason: A combination of where the psoas muscles attach and how one end of the muscle group (the torso side) is stabilized.

The iliopsoas (psoas) group attaches, on one end, to both the pelvis and the upper thigh bone. It doesn't run straight north to the sternum like the rectus abdominus, however. It runs diagonally upward and backward toward the spinal column, attaching to nearly one-third the length of the column. Close your eyes and picture yourself in a supine position on the floor. Visualize a muscle that attaches to the hip end of the thigh bone and the top and inside surfaces of the pelvic bones, then runs down towards the floor, attaching to the spinal column from its southernmost tip (the coccyx) to the mid-back. Hold the image—that's the iliopsoas.

Here's the bottom line to the story: when your feet are anchored in a Sit-Up you are *biomechanically* allowing the psoas muscles to pull your torso up *by pulling on your spine.* With the lower body anchored at the feet, the psoas contracts and forces the unstabilized end, the spine, to move. While the rectus abdominus is also working to raise the torso, the psoas is wreaking havoc on the back, pulling with great force, altering the normal, healthy, built-in curvature, and doing imperceptible but cumulative damage.

And the Leg Lift! Keep in mind that a muscle creates motion by pulling on its unanchored side. Which muscles run from the thigh to the torso, holding the legs aloft because their other attachment, the torso, is stabilized? Only two: the rectus femoris, one of the four upper thigh muscles (the quadriceps group), and our nemesis, the psoas. The rectus femoris presents no problem, for it runs from the thigh to the front of the torso and leaves the spinal column alone. The psoas, however, keeps the legs up because its *other* attachment, the spinal column, is being held stationary on the floor. Or is it?

That's right. Your back arches when you do Leg Lifts! The arch is caused by the psoas muscles pulling on the spinal column, which *cannot* easily be stabilized! And what's the net result of two heavy legs being held up by muscles that attach to the spine? Back trouble!

So why is it that the abdominal muscles feel like they're working so hard in the Leg Lift? Well, they are. But it's *not* to hold the legs up! The weight of the legs forces the pelvic girdle to rotate downward, and it's the rectus abdominus that contracts to prevent the rotation. Since the lower portion of the rectus abdominus works pretty hard, you will strengthen it through Leg Lifts. You'll also tear your lower back apart. Period. No debate.

Solution Number One

For those of you who bought just the Back Machine, and for your friends, family, and acquaintances who also are *sans* Abdominal Machine, you have an alternative. It's so simple, and so quickly verified by test, that you'll be shocked. It's called the *Unanchored-Foot Curl-Up*.

Find your way to your normal Sit-Up location and anchor your feet. Do a few Sit-Ups to get a feel for the stress they put on the abdominals and make sure to feel—with your hands—how hard the tops of the thighs are working. Now scoot out from your anchor position and try the unanchored-foot version. Place the feet flat on the floor, keep the knees elevated, and place your heels 12–18 inches from your buttocks. Close your hands into fists, then place them alongside your ears; *do not* grasp the back of your head. Begin the Curl-Up by tucking your chin into your chest, then gradually roll your torso up off the floor, *stopping when your shoulder blades leave the floor.* Hold this position for a second or two, then slowly uncurl back onto the floor.

Feel any harder? You bet! Try a few and compare how much tougher they are on the rectus abdominus, and how much less the thighs are working, than with Anchored-Foot Sit-Ups. The reason? The action of the psoas muscles and the rectus femoris, which previously took some of the load off the abdominals, has been almost entirely removed by unanchoring the feet!

But I'm getting ahead of myself. The point here is not to give you an abdominal program (that's in Chapter 7). It's to educate you as to what's wrong with what you and everyone else has been doing and why there are now $500 alternatives!

The Problem with Solution Number One

Well, we've solved the psoas problem and have increased the work load on the rectus abdominus, but we haven't provided a means for "systematic progression of intensity." In simpler words, what do we do to increase the challenge to the abdominals once they can comfortably perform 50 Curl-Ups?

The least expensive, and not terribly difficult, option is to purchase a set of dumbbells or weight plates and hold them on your chest as you curl up. This would add to the weight of your torso, and you could progressively increase the challenge. The problem? Those abdominals can get pretty strong. How strong? For those of you who already own the Abdominal Machine, and for those who can try one in a store, just try moving the pin down the range of holes one at a time. You'll be very surprised.

Solution Number Two

What if we created a machine that allowed the abdominal muscles to contract forcefully and safely but also offered ten levels of resistance? Great idea—and it's been done for the home. Granted, it's not inexpensive. But it works. The Nautilus Home Abdominal Machine solves many of the problems with existing exercise strategies for the middle.

Solves *many* of the problems? What do you mean *many*? Refer back to Figure 1, because your answer is there. A trim middle depends on more than the rectus abdominus. Three other muscles, which are *not* as perfectly stressed by the abdominal machine, help flatten the stomach. The external and internal obliques run diagonally from the sides into the midline of the abdomen, the externals running primarily downward and the internals upward and across. The transverse abdominus runs horizontally, from the sides of the torso into the midline. As noted in Chapter 1, they combine to form a natural girdle in a cross-your-stomach configuration.

To help you sculpt a truly statuesque middle, the Total Torso

Program will include a special exercise or two to focus on the obliques and transverse abdominus. But we're not quite there yet. That's Chapter 7.

THE PROBLEMS WITH BACK EXERCISES

If you think it's tough to train the abdominals, wait 'til you try the back! And now that you're an expert anatomist (see Figure 2 on page 19) and biomechanist, it won't take long to show you why.

There are two main problems. The first, discussed earlier, is range of motion. You should remember that maximal results require that muscles be trained through their full range of motion. That's a tough request for back extension exercises but one that *can* be met. The more difficult problem is the need for progressive resistance—making the exercise harder as your lower back strengthens. That's a nearly impossible order to fill in the best of the nonmachine back exercises.

Please take note here: nowhere is it irrefutably established that, the stronger your back gets, the less your chances of back trouble. Besides being a logical conclusion, though, there is early research support for the idea that back extensor strength and endurance are related to lower back health. (The extensors, by the way, seen in Figure 2, are the muscles that run from the pelvic girdle to the torso. With the pelvis stabilized, they move the torso backward, in a motion called *extension.*)

A fascinating study of the lower back by Swedish researcher Finn Sorenson recently won the internationally recognized Volvo Award for excellence. Sorenson gave all 1,000 residents of a small Swedish town a battery of tests to assess the health, strength, and endurance of their lower backs, then followed them for one year. At the end of the period, he remeasured the people and correlated his test results with any incidences of back problems.

Sorenson found that the test that best predicted whether someone was going to have back problems was a simple isometric hold in the Back Extension position. Each subject climbed onto a tabletop in a prone position, then extended the head and torso out over the edge. With a spotter holding their lower bodies firmly to the table, they extended far

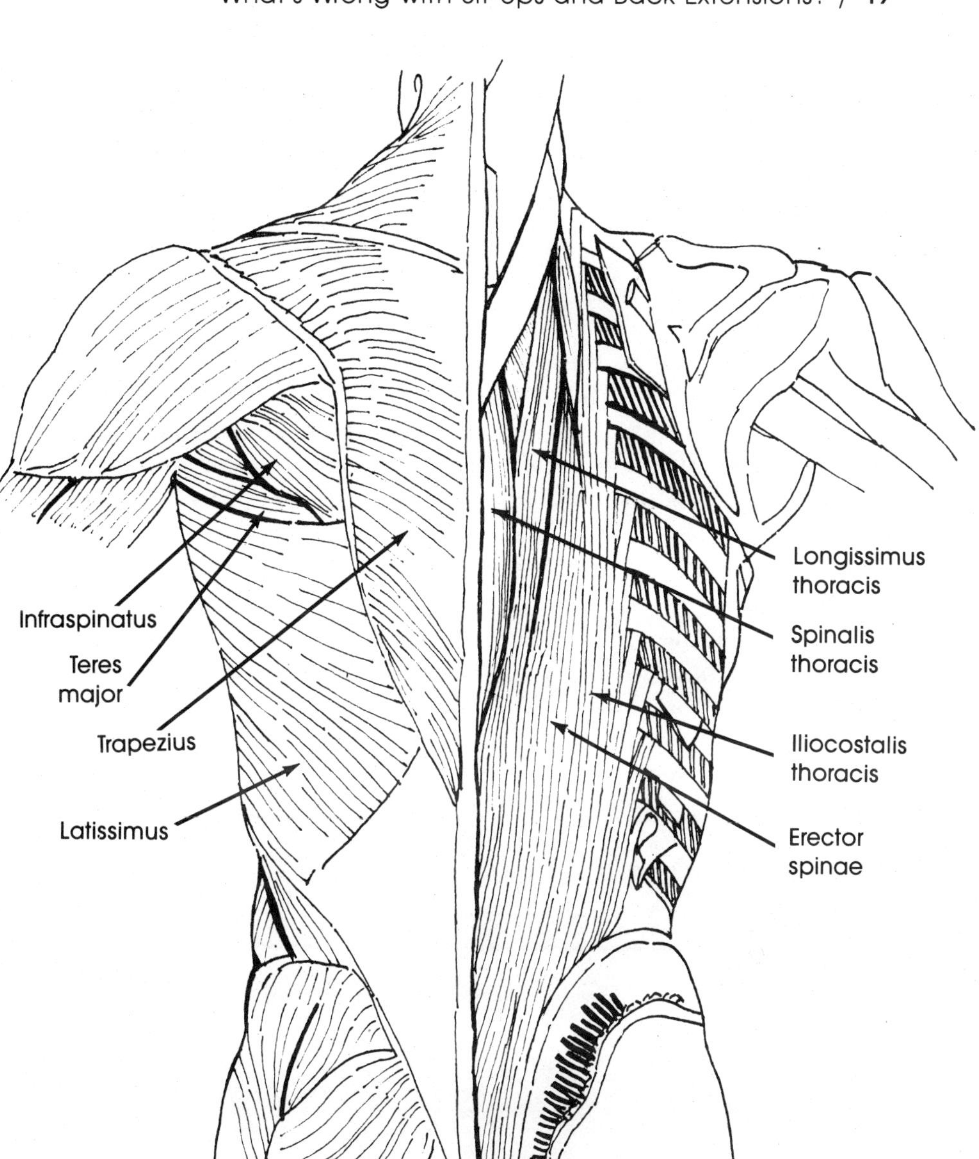

Primary muscles of the back (the Back Extensors).

enough over the edge to be able to bend freely from the waist toward the floor. The test required that the subject elevate the head and torso to a position parallel with the floor (a straight line from head to toe), then hold motionless as long as possible. The maximum time was set at 240 seconds. Sorenson found that the people who had the longest isometric (motionless) hold times in pretesting were those least likely to suffer back problems during the year.

Now, how does this affect you at home? If you didn't buy the Back Machine, Chapter 5 will show you how to adapt Sorenson's isometric test to make it a dynamic (moving) exercise. Pictured is a Back Extension off the floor, which is considerably less difficult. You'll also get instructions on performing Extensions off a tabletop.

I got off on this semitangent because I told you that it was nearly impossible to create a progressive resistance exercise for the lower back extensors. You could do it off a tabletop holding dumbbells in your hands, but, having tried it, I'm not very confident about recommending it to anyone! The option that you and many people are choosing is the Nautilus Home Back Machine, which offers ten levels of resistance and a very nice range of motion.

4

USING YOUR NAUTILUS MACHINES

THE NATURE OF THE BEAST

For those of you familiar with the Nautilus philosophy of training to the point of momentary muscular failure, you're in for a slightly different program here. Because of the nature of the muscles involved, you won't be shooting for 12–15 repetitions. Nautilus advises 40 for the home machines, based on the fact that your abs and back extensors are categorized as *slow-twitch,* or *red,* muscles.

Briefly stated, human muscle is found in four categories that are based on both behavior and chemistry. The three fast and powerfully contracting fiber types are called, not surprisingly, *fast-twitch muscles.* (A twitch is one rapid contraction of a fiber.) The one category that contracts more slowly and with less force is called *slow-twitch.*

Why does this all matter? It matters more than you might think, affecting *all* your strength training. It turns out that only fast-twitch muscles respond to strength training with significant size increases. Slow-twitch muscle can get stronger, but it rarely gets bigger. Now you know why some of your muscles seem to grow while others don't. It's not necessarily the machine or the exercise—the percentages of slow and fast muscle fibers are genetically fixed and different for every muscle. While your deltoids (shoulders) might be 80 percent fast-twitch, your front thighs (quadriceps) might be 80 percent slow-twitch. In my own case, my chest (pectoralis), deltoids, and middle back (latissimus) grow almost at the mere thought of strength training, while my quadriceps and biceps get very strong but never get big. It's very likely a result of fiber type percentages.

In the case of the abdomen and back, the muscles are almost totally composed of slow-twitch fibers. This has two implications. First, you do not have to be afraid of growing large muscles in these areas. Second, and more importantly, you will most likely get greater benefits from higher repetitions, since the slow-twitch fibers are also high in endurance. They need a longer stimulus—e.g., 40 reps instead of 12—to strengthen maximally. And since they will get stronger but not bigger, the net result is a tighter, trimmer figure.

Why 40 repetitions and not 50? There's no way at this early point in the machines' history to know if 50 might be several percent better, or if 30 might be the optimal number. I have no problem going along with the 40-rep advice. And remember, just as with commercial Nautilus equipment, that suggested number of repetitions is the exact point at which you should reach momentary muscular failure. Should you get to 40 and find that you have the wherewithal for six more reps before the muscles say no, do 'em!

What's this nonsense about momentary muscular failure, Nautilus novices ask? Simply, working to the point at which the muscles can no longer create sufficient force to contract leaves nothing to chance. No guessing at what 80 percent intensity means. No guessing about two or three sets of estimated 75 percent intensity. What has worked spectacularly through fifteen years of Nautilus is the simple advice to perform only one set of each strength training exercise and always to work to the point of momentary muscular failure.

GENERAL PRINCIPLE 1:
Aim for momentary muscular failure at the 40-repetition point, but continue working if you don't fail.

THE SPEED OF TRAINING ISSUE

S - L - O - W. If that's not clear enough, follow this rule: slow when performing the concentric or positive contraction (forward on the Abdominal Machine, backward on the Back Machine) and *slower* on the negative or eccentric phase. In hard numbers, the concentric phase should take you about four seconds and the eccentric about six. Why so slow? You definitely don't want the scientific dissertation on that, so let's just say that it's safer and more effective.

GENERAL PRINCIPLE 2:
The concentric phase of each rep should last about four seconds, the eccentric phase about six.

THE PROGRESSION OF TRAINING INTENSITY

There's absolutely no magic to this plan: each and every time you reach the 40-repetition goal you must increase the difficulty one level at your next workout. And please note that we're talking about 40 reps in perfect form, with not a whit of variation from the four second–six second guideline or the instructions and photos that follow in a few pages.

Before you forget: Get out a flat-head screwdriver, a set of wrenches or vise-grip pliers, and a set of hex or Allen wrenches. It's time to switch your Back Machine from the factory-preset level of difficulty to the easier one.

Using the screwdriver and vise-grip or wrench, remove the black plastic cowling from the outside of the weight stack side of the machine. This should result in the baring of the metal arm that rises out of the resistance box (with its nine numbers)

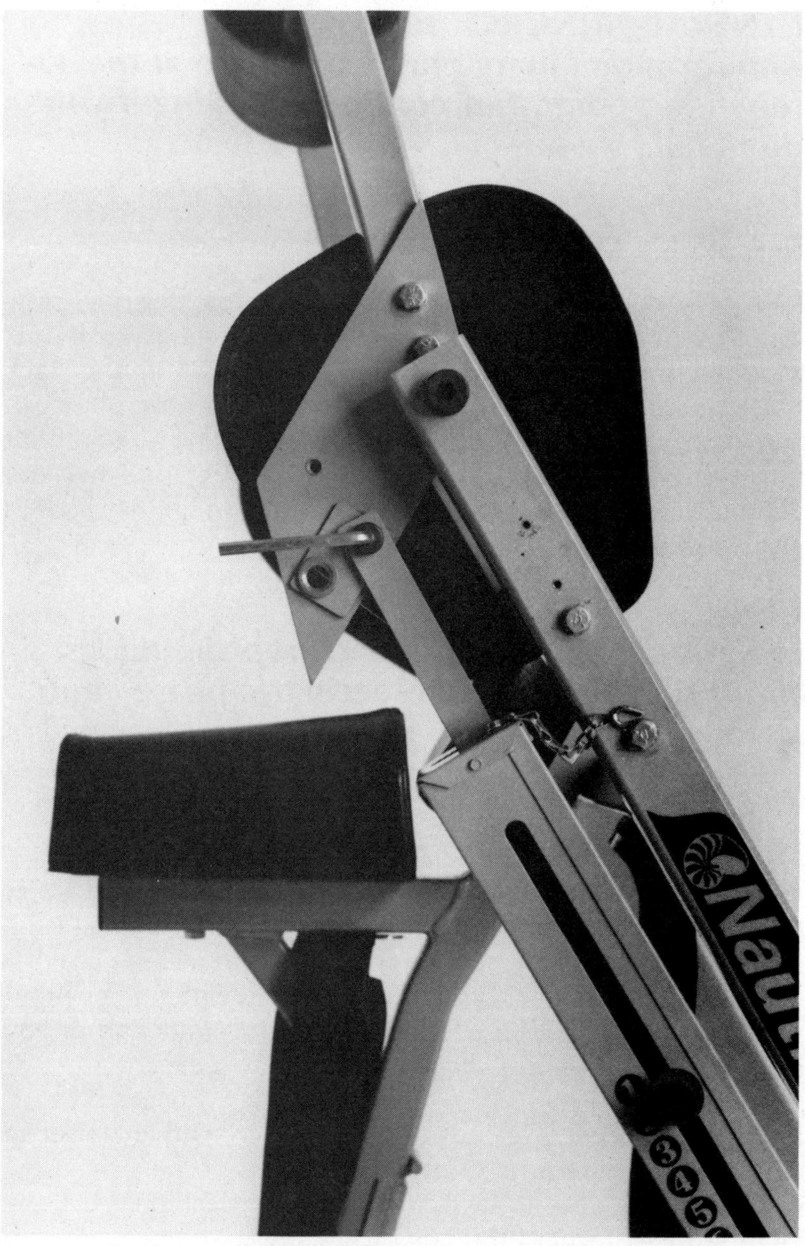

Using a "hex" or "allen" wrench to change the resistance setting on the back machine. Wrench is shown in the "B" or easier setting.

and the trapezoidal metal piece it attaches to. The attachment is a round, threaded piece with a hole in it for a six-sided wrench. These wrenches are called *hex* or *Allen wrenches,* and if you don't own a set, buy one! The fate of your back literally rides on it.

Find the hex wrench that fits snugly into the hole and remove the round nut. Maneuver the arm coming from the resistance box so that it falls over the other hole (the "B" hole), and tighten the nut in place. Replace the cowling and move on.

STARTING OFF AT THE TOP

If you haven't already established your correct intensity settings through trial and error, begin with the pin out of the machine, which Nautilus calls level 1. Following instructions to the letter, perform as many repetitions as possible in perfect form until you reach momentary muscular failure or until you feel any unusual pain in the abdomen or back. Should you reach 40 on day one, fine. Wait 48 hours, then place the pin in the first set of holes, which we now know is level 2. Shoot for 40 reps in perfect form, but remember to continue past 40 if you have the energy. If you succeed, level 3 is next up in 48 hours. If you fall short of 40, repeat level 2 at your next workout, and for as many workouts as necessary, until you *can* reach 40. When you reach level 9 and can do 40 reps in perfect form, call me. I want to see your body in person. Should anyone reach level 9 on the Back Machine, the switch can be made *back* to the factory intensity setting.

Now, I'm sure the gluttons for punishment or the particularly rotund among you want to know why you can't use your Abdominal Machine every day. And perhaps those with back problems, or a strong fear of impending back problems, feel the same way about the new Back Machine.

The greater the intensity of exercise, the less frequent it *should* be and, actually, the less frequent it *can* be. Strength exercise performed to momentary muscular failure is of such intensity that at least 48 hours must separate consecutive workouts. Anything less and the body is unlikely to have fully recovered and grown. The body will, in fact, let you know if you're overtraining. If you're following instructions to the letter, soreness that persists over more than the first week or a slowing or plateau in results is a good sign that you're working with too little rest. In my extensive experience with the Nautilus commercial machines, I've seen and personally trained many elite athletes who could safely strength train no more than two times a week.

GENERAL PRINCIPLE 3:
Increase the intensity level by one hole in your next workout each time you reach the 40-repetition point.

Chapter 7 will present the Total Torso Program, with details on when to do what.

THE BACK MACHINE ILLUSTRATED

I agreed to write this book for one altruistic reason. I am *convinced* that the Nautilus Home Back Machine could be dangerous if used without at least three preliminary stretches and a warm-up set of repetitions on the easiest intensity setting. Here's the way you get ready (stretched), get set (warm-up reps), and go.

Stretches

Stretch 1: Knees to Chest. From a supine position, bring both knees into the chest, grabbing below the kneecaps and exerting a gentle pull. Do not lift the lower back off the floor. Hold in a stretched position for at least 20 seconds, release to the floor, then repeat at least once.

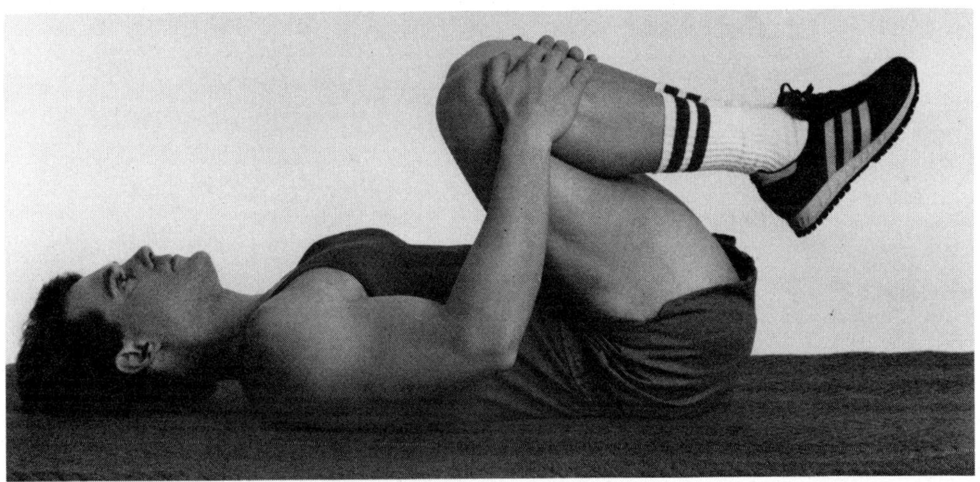

The "Knees to Chest" stretch.

Stretch 2: The Modified Yoga Plow. Done incorrectly, this can play tricks with your cervical spine, so follow closely. In a supine position, place the arms out diagonally as shown with the palms down. Lift the extended legs simultaneously overhead, only far enough to lift the lower back off the floor. Keeping the torso in this position, let the feet drop toward the floor as the muscles in the back of the thighs (the hamstrings) and the lower back relax and stretch. Hold for at least 20 seconds, slowly return the legs to starting position, then repeat once or twice more.

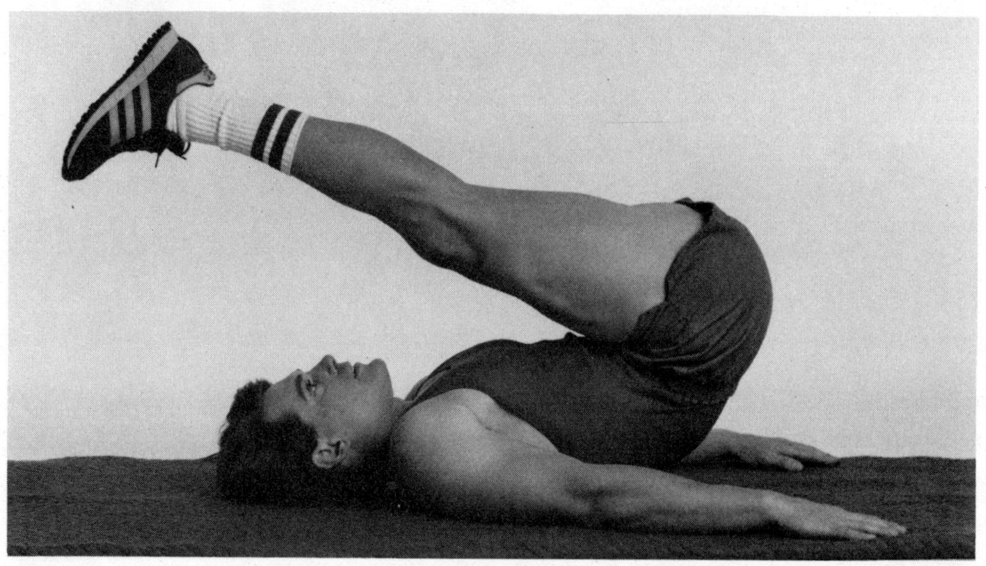

The Modified Plow.

Stretch 3: The Torso Twister. Sit upright with both legs extended in front, toes up. Cross the right foot over to the outside of the left knee. Twist the torso slowly to the right, placing the left elbow on the outside of the raised right knee. Hold this position for at least 20 seconds, relax, and repeat once more. Reverse the positions (twisting to the left side) and complete two additional 20-second stretches.

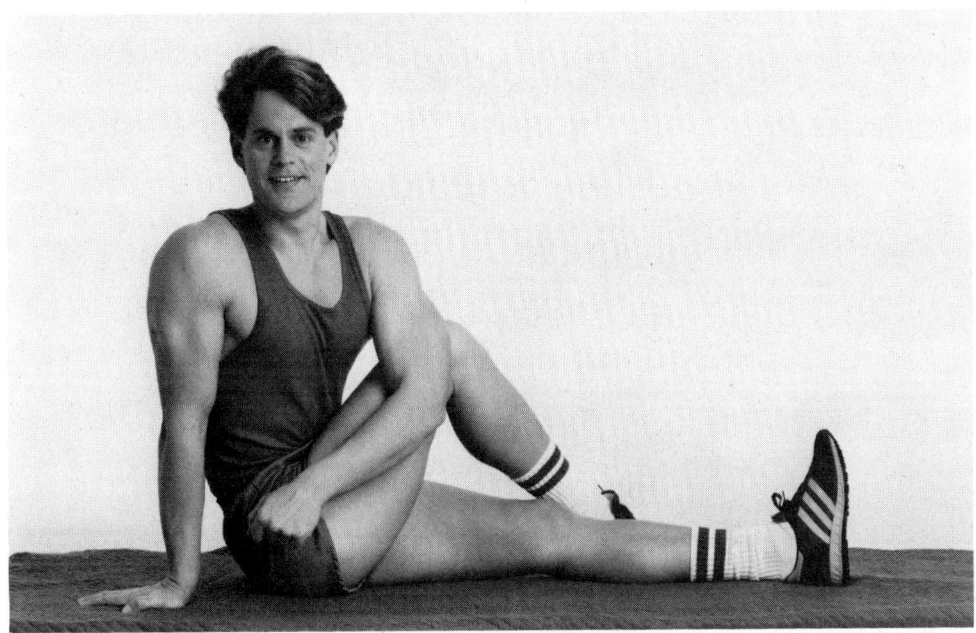

The Torso Twist.

Setting Up

Setting footrest height. No difficulties likely here. Simply raise or lower the seat to give you an approximation of the angle shown in the photo. You are welcome to experiment, but *do not* venture too close to a straight-leg position.

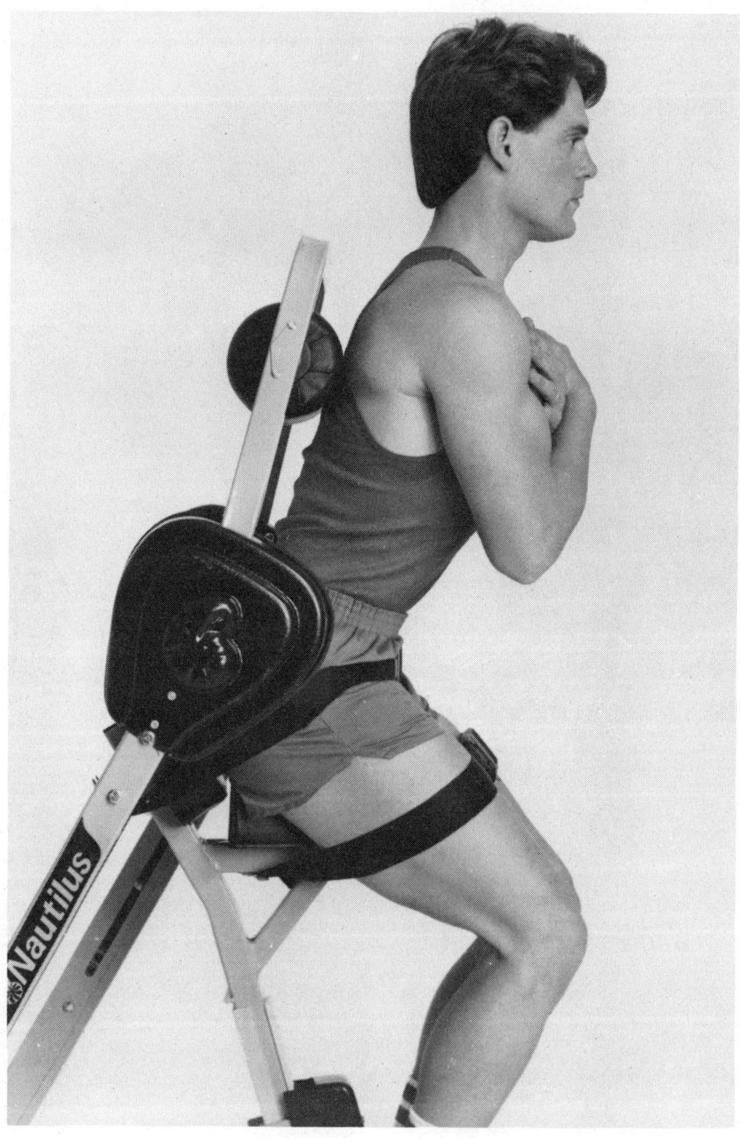

Approximate knee angle for safe use of back machine.

Setting the resistance level. Since you will *always* start with a warm-up set, remove the pin from the machine. Shown below is the second level, with the pin somewhere between numbers 1 and 2. Remember "pin out of machine" for level 1 intensity, "pin in first hole" for level 2.

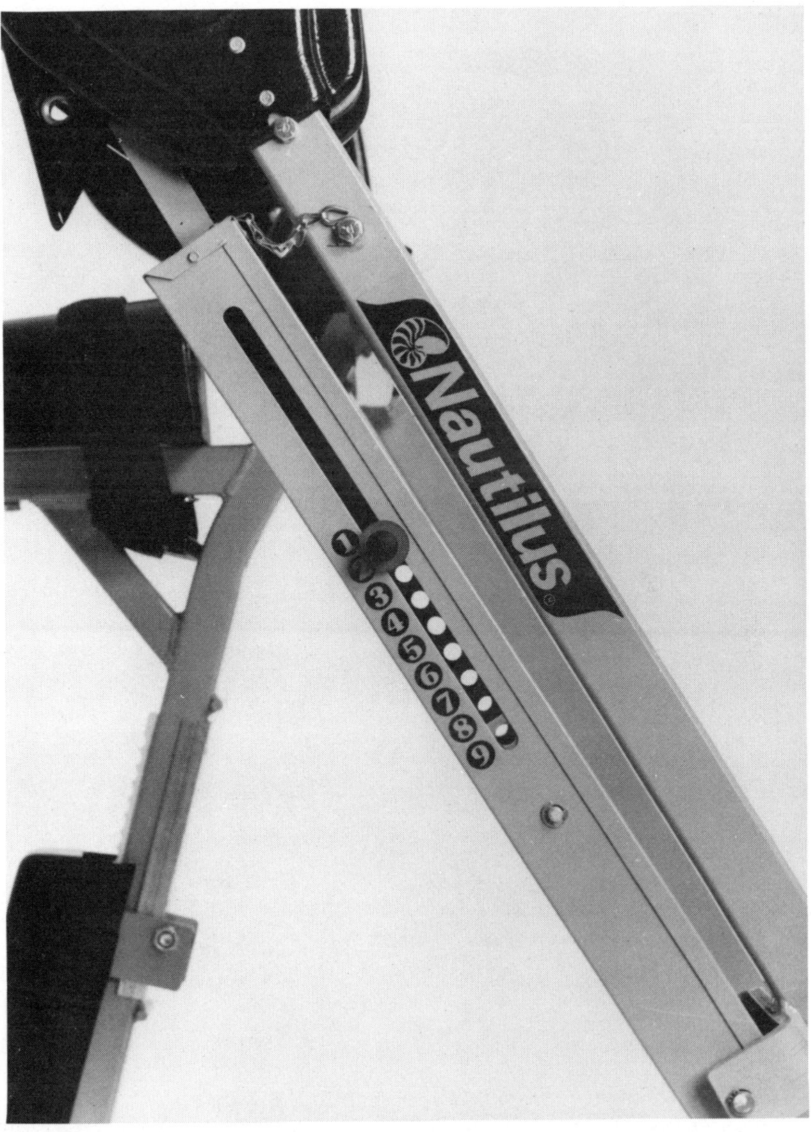

Pin shown in first set of holes, which yields the second level of resistance.

How not to change the pin. Never attempt to lean around the machine to change the resistance level while strapped in. Both home machines are poorly balanced and will easily tip over if you try this maneuver. *Be careful.*

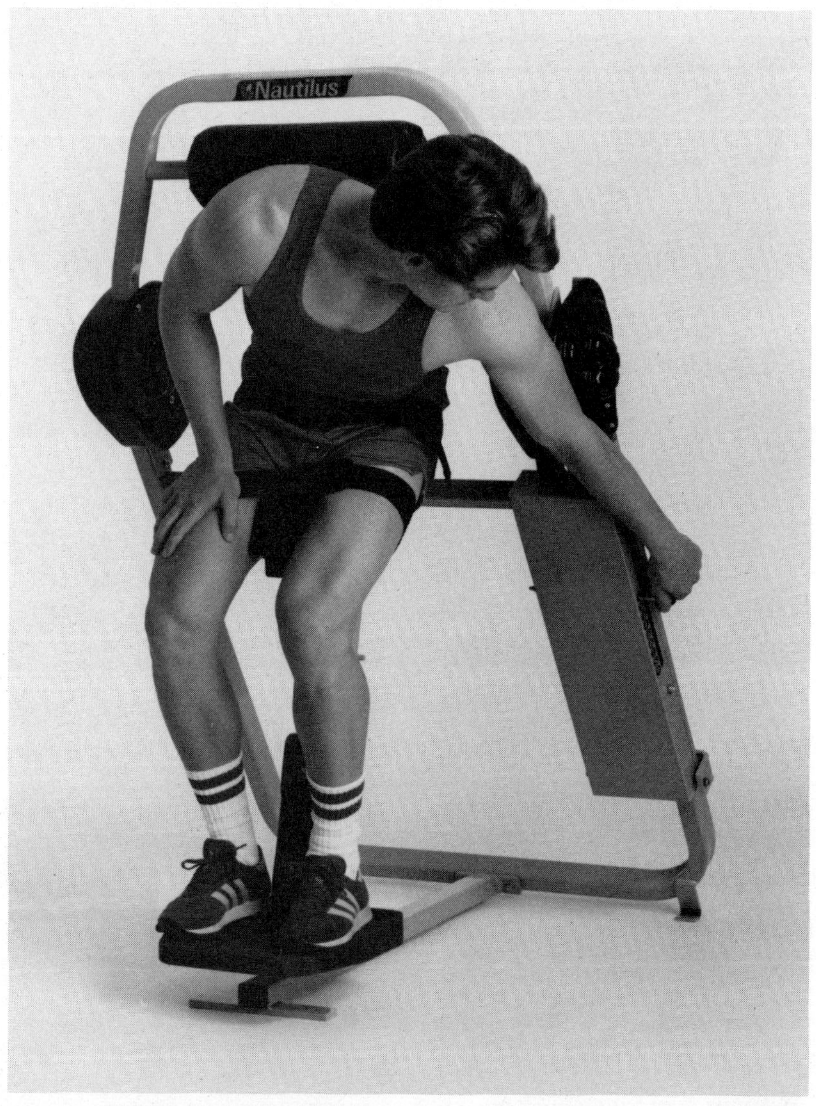

How ***not*** *to change the pin. Do not lean to the weight stack side while strapped into the machine.*

The Warm-Up Set

Regardless of how strong you are and what level you're going to train at, I strongly recommend a warm-up set of 20 repetitions. The back is obviously an area not to be toyed with. The resistances on the Home Back Machine are extremely high, even at level 2 or 3. I mean it. Warm-up comes first!

Go!

Starting position. After setting the correct footrest height, keep the heels at the back of the rest and strap in as tightly as possible. Take me literally here—the belts are the anchor we talked about earlier that lets the back extensors work. I really mean *as tightly as possible*. The arms may be crossed, may rest on the thighs, or may be used for assistance as shown below.

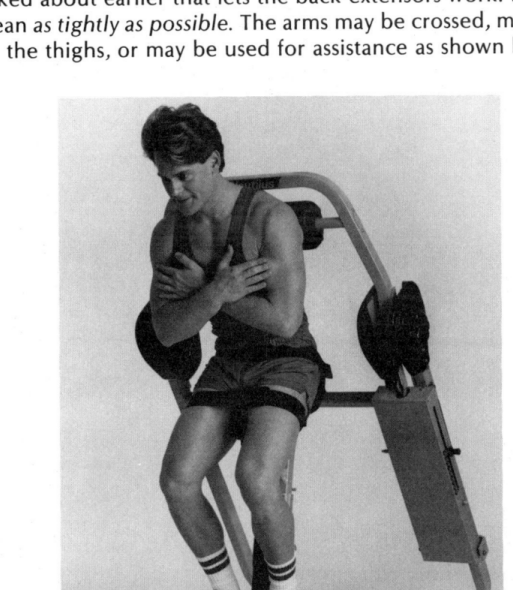

Starting position, Back Machine.

For those who have trouble at level 1. The first two women who tried the Back Machine after I set it up had trouble at level 2. Shown below is the solution: spotting yourself with your hands. From the starting position, move both hands back behind the horizontal bar with the palms facing forward. You can now use the muscles in your arms and shoulders to assist the back extensors. This is not a permanent fix. It is intended to give your back that little boost of help so that it can be challenged at higher intensity levels, rather than get permanently stuck at a lower level. Try to wean yourself off this trick as your back strengthens.

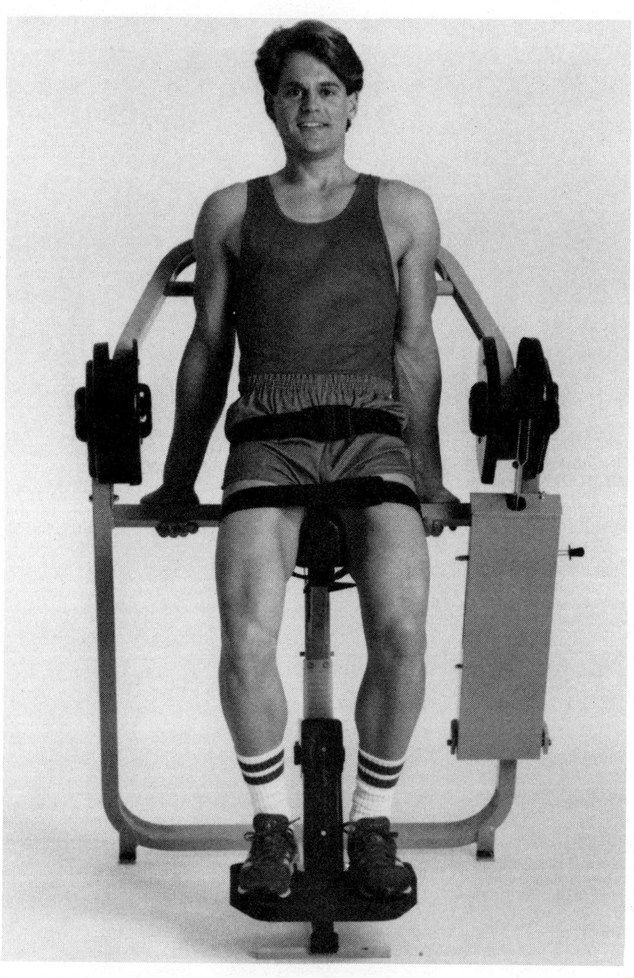

Using the arms to assist the back extensor muscles. Anyone having difficulty completing the movement at level 1 should try this option. It is not to be used in cases of simple fatigue.

Remember to move slowly! Take about four seconds to extend smoothly backward, starting with a *smooth* application of force rather than a burst. Contract until you reach the end of the range of motion and hold this position isometrically (motionless) for a count of two. Take about six seconds to return to the starting position. Pause only momentarily, then continue. Repeat to momentary muscular failure, which should occur at about 40 repetitions.

Discontinue the exercise at the slightest indication of unusual pain. Muscle cramps may be relieved through massage and/or heat. If any pain persists hours after the exercise, or if you experience any feelings of numbness or tingling in the legs consult a physician.

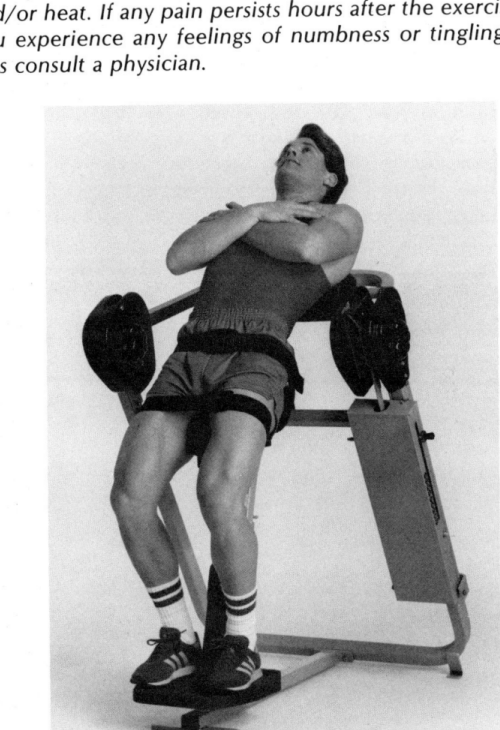

Finish position, Back Machine.

THE ABDOMINAL MACHINE ILLUSTRATED

Since the abdominal region is less sensitive to insult and trauma than the lower back, you won't need to go through quite the same preparation as you did for the first machine. As is true of all intense exercise, though, you should not undertake it without at least some warm-up.

Those of you who've already used the Abdominal Machine know that it *is* stressful on the lower back. I strongly suggest that you precede your Abdominal Machine work with at least two of the three stretches shown earlier (pages 27–29). I don't feel a warm-up set of repetitions is necessary, however.

Setting Up

Setting seat height. Get to know the seat adjustment operation and get into the habit of always checking that the seat is firmly in place before jumping on. Note how the seat is tilted up to allow positioning. I have seen a six-month pregnant woman forget to check the security of the seat position on a Nautilus shoulder machine and go crashing to the floor.

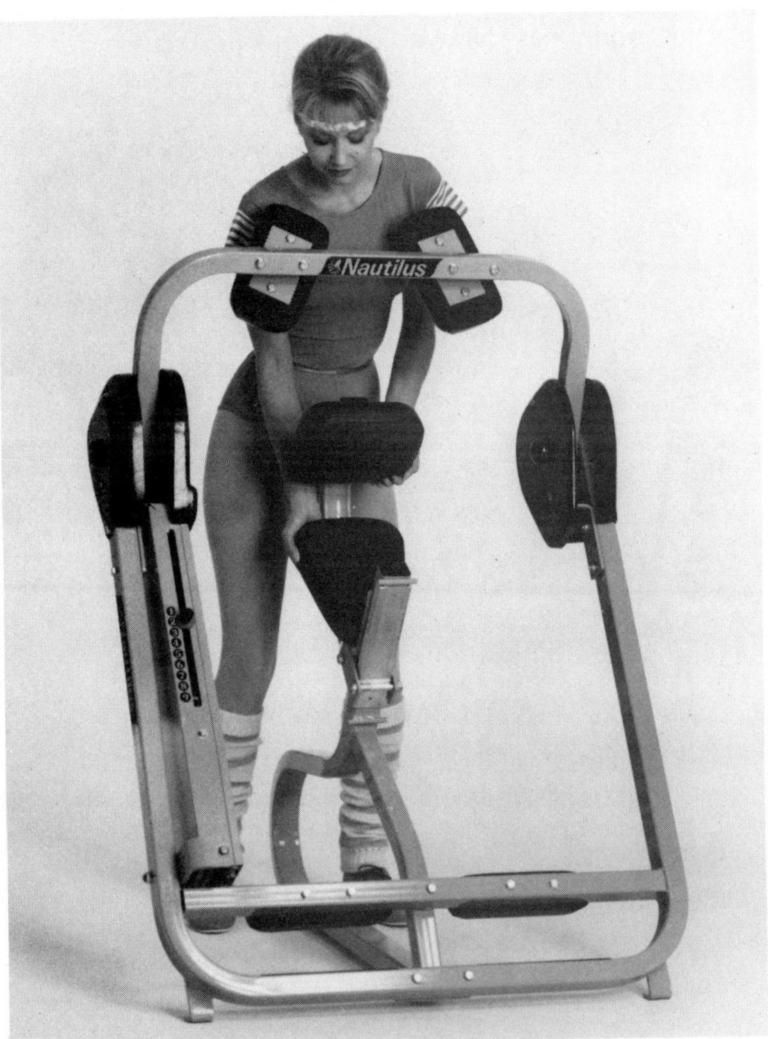

Setting the seat height on the Abdominal Machine. Tilt the back of the seat up and slide the whole assembly into position.

Matching torso and machine axes. Stand outside the machine, and with the pin out, swing the horizontal bar forward. Note its "axis of rotation," the point around which it rotates. (It's a round protrusion in the middle of the black plastic cowling.)

Now bend forward from your waist and make a mental note of *your* axis of rotation, which is roughly the hip joint. Your goal in setting seat height on the machine is to match the machine's axis with your axis. Note in the close-up (below) that the model has followed directions perfectly!

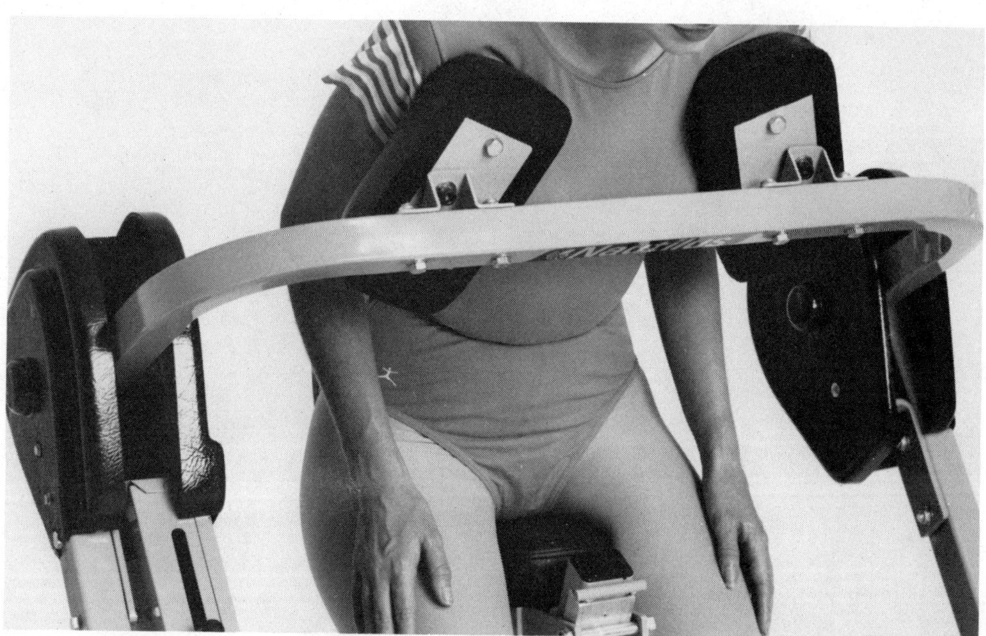

Closeup of the matching of torso and machine axes of rotation. The knob on the black plastic cowling matches the axis around which the torso bends forward.

Reminders. *Do not* attempt to adjust the resistance while seated in the machine. Since you're not strapped in, just get out and do it right. Also, level 1 resistance is set with the pin *out* of the machine, level 2 with the pin in the first hole.

Climbing in. Standing to one side of the seat, which you have checked, place both hands on the horizontal bar and push it forward (if possible) to ease entry. Lift one leg over the seat and climb in. Possible hitch: you may dislodge the seat from its secure position as you lift the leg over. I have seen this happen!

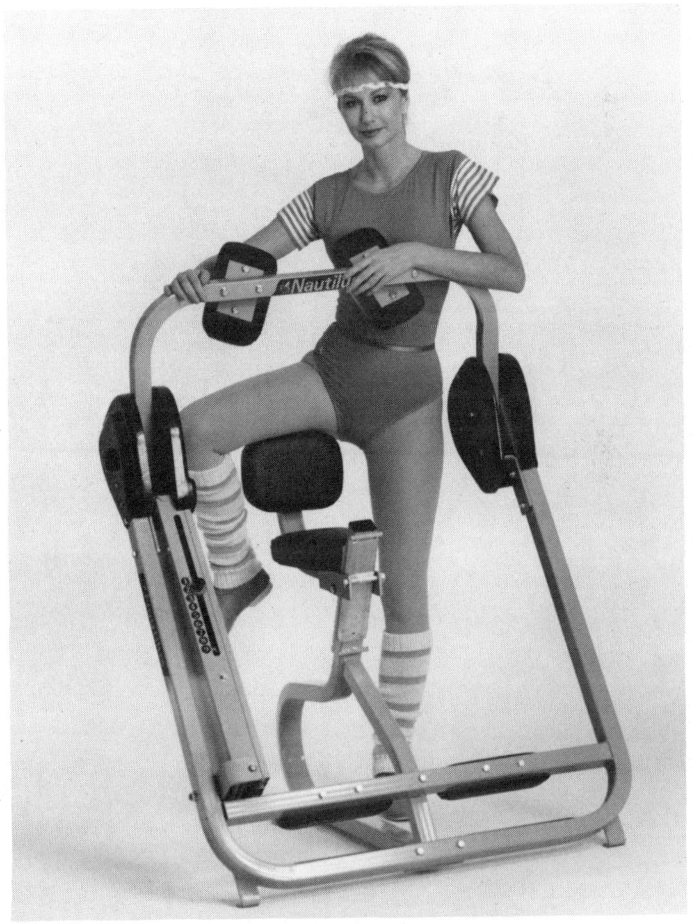

Climbing into the machine. Check that the seat is firmly in place; hold the horizontal arm forward and out of the way.

Go!

Starting position. Wedge your toes in between the bottom two horizontal bars and rotate the shoulder pads around until they feel comfortable. The hands may rest on the thighs or be placed in any unobtrusive position. You can even try holding closed fists up at the sides of your head, as in the Curl-Up described earlier.

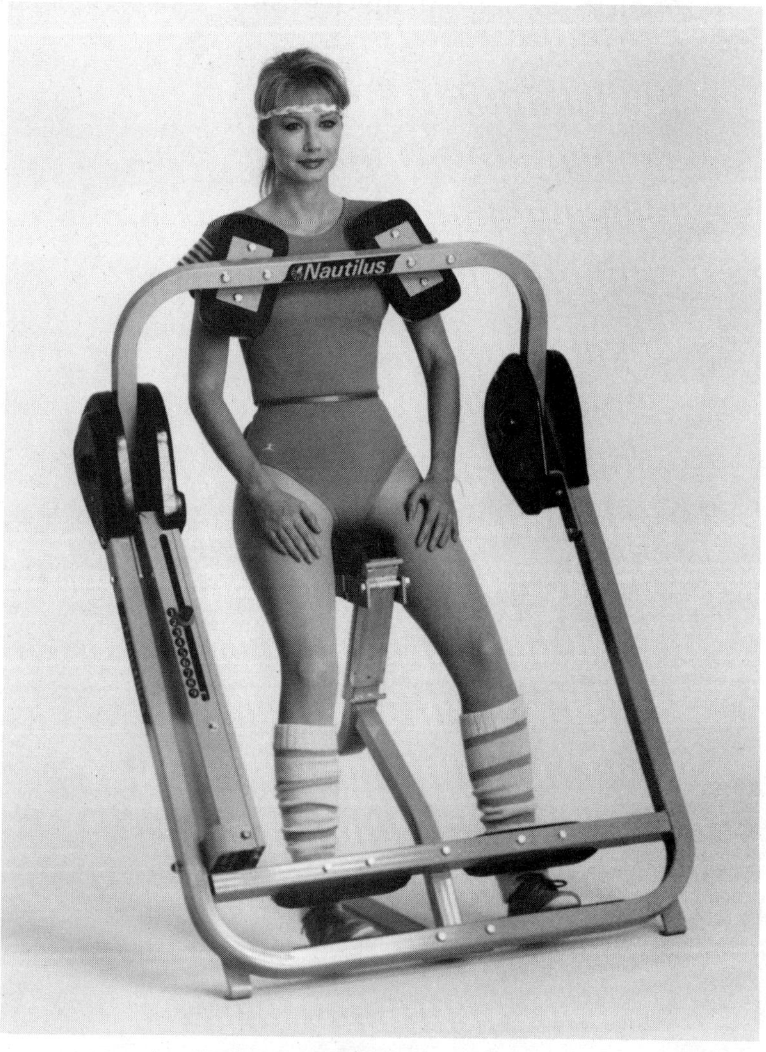

Starting position, Abdominal Machine.

Remember to move slowly! Begin the movement with a slow application of force. *Do not* explode into the pads like some crazed football lineman. Make sure you are firmly planted all the way back on the seat. The knees should remain comfortably apart. Round the back slightly as you curl forward, keeping the head down and moving in about four seconds' time to the end of the machine's range of motion. Hold this fully contracted position for about two seconds, then return in about six seconds' time to the starting position. Pause only momentarily (or not at all) there, then repeat. The goal is momentary muscular failure at the 40th perfect repetition. Continue beyond 40 if the will and energy are there. Should you fall short of 40, continue at that resistance level in following workouts until the goal is reached. Remember, it is more valuable for you to do 37 reps in perfect form than 45 sloppily.

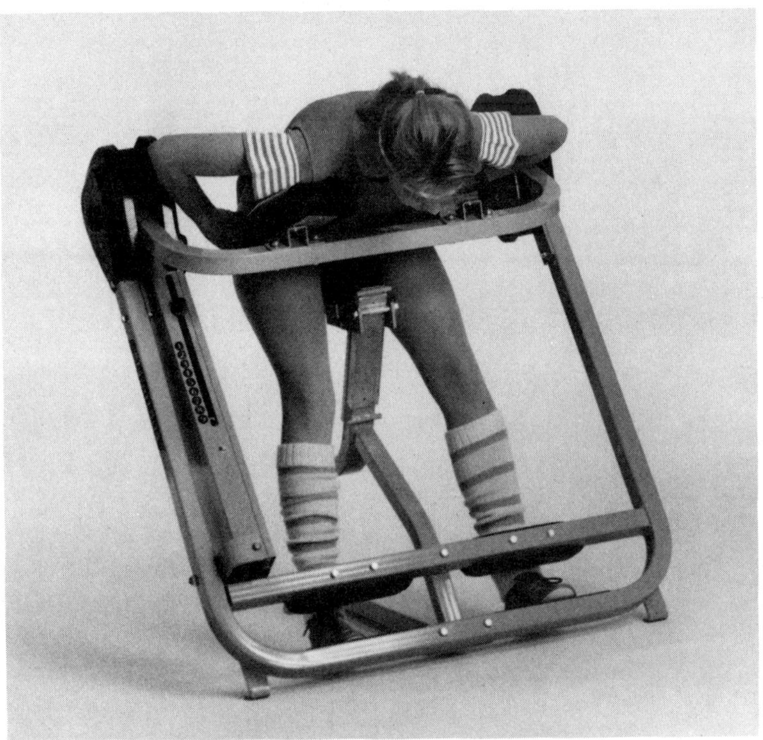

Finish position, Abdominal Machine.

FOR THOSE WHO ARE WONDERING . . .

If you do own both machines and are anxious to start on a program at this time before reading on, here's a preview: Your best bet is to use the machines on alternate days. Abdominal work might be on a Monday-Wednesday-Friday schedule, and back work on a Tuesday-Thursday-Saturday shift. I don't recommend doing both on the same day.

5

SUPPLEMENTING YOUR NAUTILUS HOME MACHINES

As I noted earlier, the muscles of your torso are responsible for far more than bending you in both directions. The muscles that rotate the torso, primarily the internal and external obliques and the transverse abdominus, all need to be trained for truly total torso integrity. They *do* receive some benefit from the flexion movement of the Abdominal Machine and the extension of the Back Machine, however.

As I also noted earlier, many of you have purchased only one of the two machines. The exercises below will go far toward training that region of your torso not fortunate enough to have a machine of its own. Some instructions on putting your program together are presented here; complete instructions for combining machine work with these exercises are presented in Chapter 7.

TRAINING THE OBLIQUES, TRANSVERSE ABS, AND LOWER ABS

I've chosen several of my favorite abdominal exercises to show you here based on their effectiveness at training the muscles not optimally worked by the Abdominal Machine. The Side Leg Throw, and eventually its advanced variation, should be performed after each set on your Abdominal Machine. Those of you without the Abdominal Machine will work with these exercises:

- Basic Curl-Up (Chapter 3)
- Side Leg Throw, progressing to Assisted Leg Throw
- Basic Leg Exchange, progressing to Leg Exchange with Torso Twist

The latter two will be shown and described here; the Total Torso Program that incorporates them is found in Chapter 7.

Keeping the feet together, throw the legs to one side (using leg power, not your hands), stopping them before they reach the floor. The lower back may raise slightly. Hold this position only momentarily; then, using the muscles in the outer hip and outer thigh of the top leg, lift the still-straight legs back to the starting position. Pause, then repeat the movement to the other side. Begin with as few repetitions as you can comfortably perform and progress by adding one repetition per workout. When you can perform 30 reps to each side, you might move to the advanced variation described below.

The Side Leg Throw. From a supine position, with your arms spread to the sides for balance, lift both legs to a vertical position as shown. Toes should be comfortably pointed, feet together. Men with tight hamstrings who are having a tough time keeping the legs straight should just do the best they can. (Hamstring stretching is in order.)

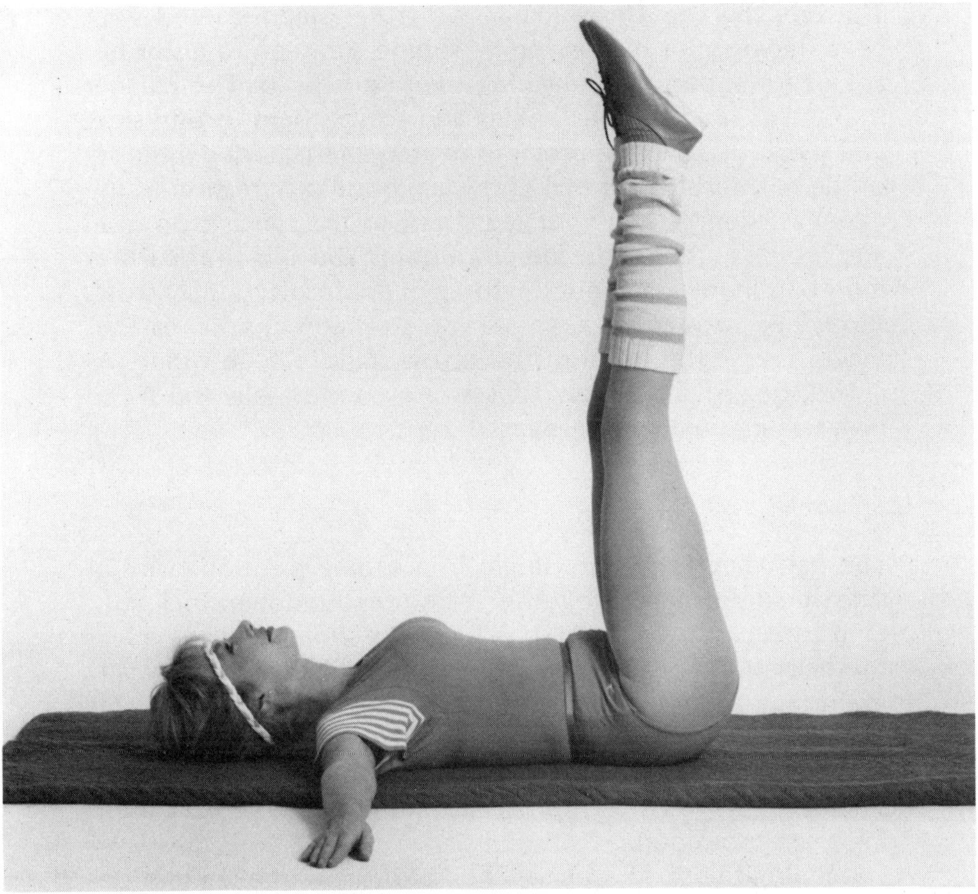

Starting position, Leg Throws.

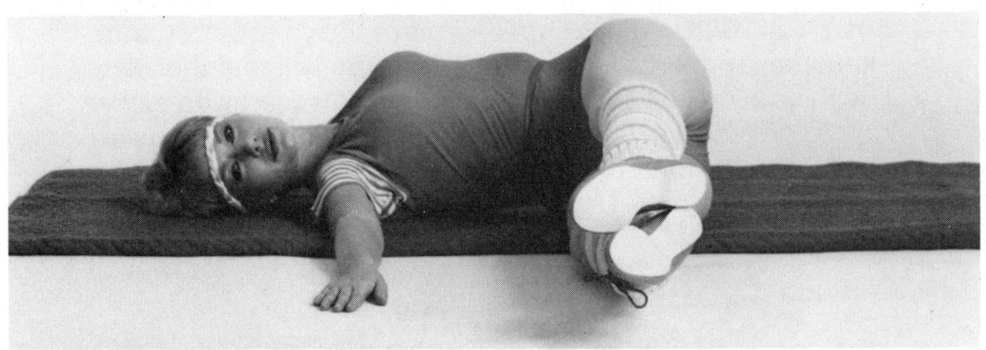

Finish position, Leg Throws.

The Assisted Leg Throw. Have a partner stand behind your head, facing your feet as you lie supine. Hold on to his or her ankles for support by reaching over your head. The partner then takes hold of your ankles and tosses them to one side, and you resist as in the previous exercise. (The added intensity of the partner's throw makes this a natural progression to the easier version.) Draw your legs back to the starting position and repeat to the other side. *Important:* You and your partner *must* communicate about the force of the throw. Initial throws should be of low intensity; as you strengthen, your partner may increase the force of the throw. Talk to each other! As above, begin with as few reps as are comfortable and try to progress gradually to perhaps 30 reps.

The Basic Leg Exchange. Begin in a supine position, arms at side, head down, legs together, toes pointed down. Tuck your chin and curl the torso up so that *just the shoulder blades* clear the floor. Arms reach forward, elevated slightly. It is *critically* important that your torso remain elevated, for it prevents damage to the lower back from the psoas, which does some of the work in exchanging the legs. (Raising the torso as shown stabilizes the pelvis and spinal column, preventing back arching from psoas pull.)

Keeping the torso, outstretched arms, and one leg motionless, bring the other leg up and into the chest while bending at the knee (halfway point is pictured). Hamstring flexibility will determine how close you can get the knee to the chest; do the best you can. Now extend this leg while drawing the other, outstretched leg up and into the chest. Continue alternating in a bicycling-type motion. You will feel the exercise in both the lower and upper abdominals. Start with as few reps as are comfortable, progressing to 100 (each knee-to-chest counts as one rep).

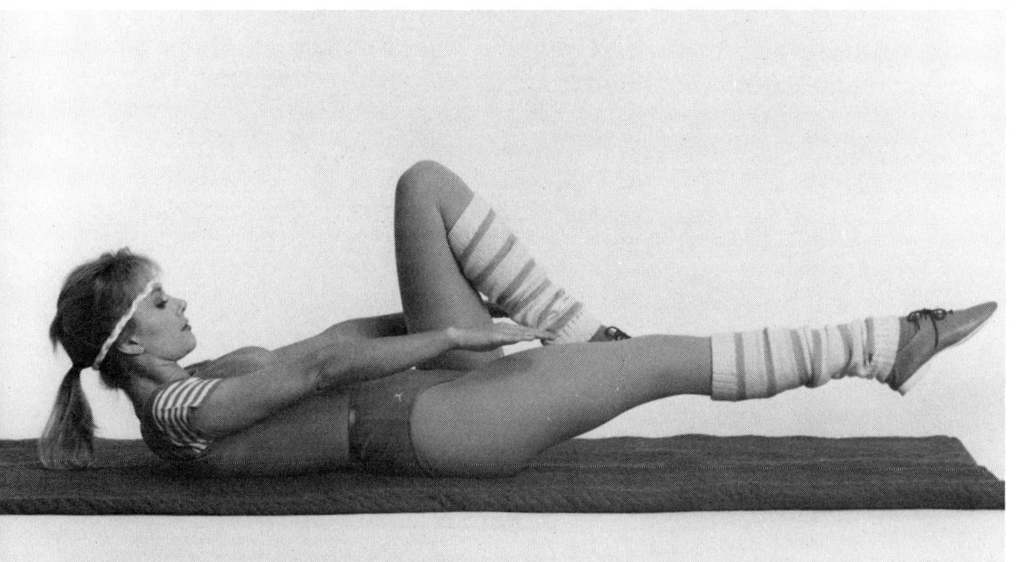

Up position, Leg Exchange (basic version).

Leg Exchange with Torso Twist. Once you reach 100 reps of the basic version you can progress to this winner. Begin in the same position: supine, legs extended, torso lifted slightly off floor. Bring the closed fists to the sides of the head and draw one of the legs up as earlier. Twist the torso so that the right elbow touches the left knee, then exchange legs as earlier and touch the left elbow to the right knee. The torso remains aloft through the entire exercise. Start with a comfortable number of reps and progress to 100. This exercise trains the whole team: upper, lower, and transverse abdominals and the internal and external obliques.

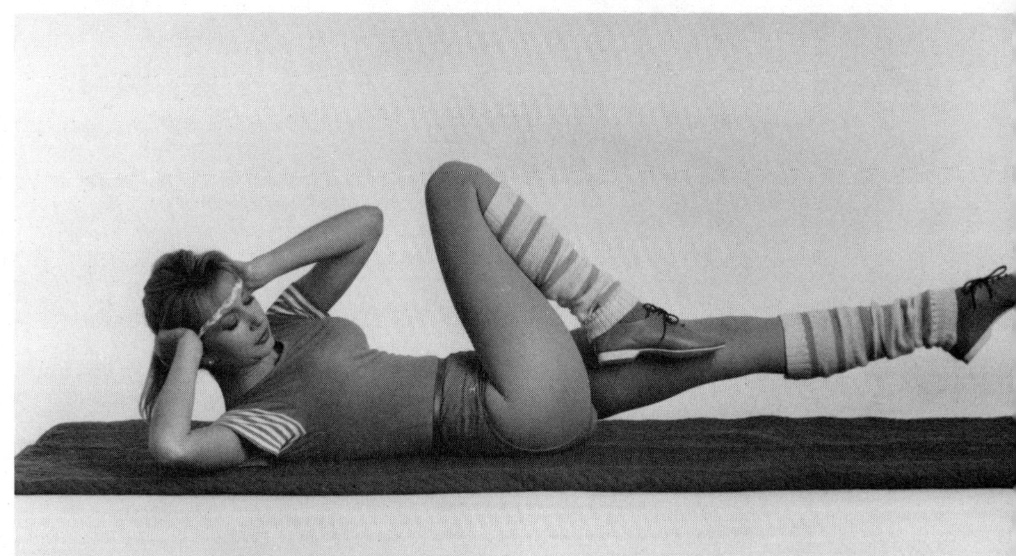

Up position, Leg Exchange (advanced version).

TRAINING THE BACK EXTENSORS

If you own only the Abdominal Machine, these exercises are for you. Besides the difficulty and potential safety problems inherent in training the rotators of the back, it's not entirely necessary if you really shape up the entire abdominal team. Those of you who *do* own the Back Machine can skip right ahead to Chapter 6.

The Basic Back Extension. This is the easier version of the two extension exercises and should be attempted first. It requires a spotter to stabilize your lower body. With your hands held at the head, or with a comfortable variation of that position, raise the torso slowly—starting at the neck and progressing down the back—to approximately the height shown. Those of you with young, healthy, pain-free backs may reach higher, but *no one* should arch the back excessively to gain height. If you *are* that fit, you'll likely reach the 40-repetition goal quickly and be ready for the advanced version.

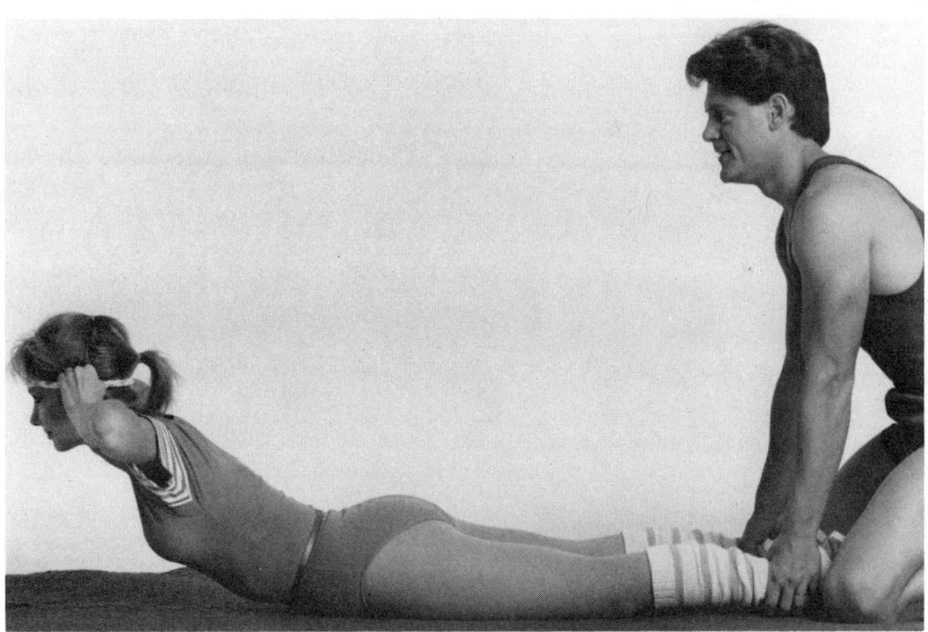

Back Extension off floor with spotter.

Advanced Back Extensions. As described in Chapter 3, a full range of motion in this exercise can be obtained by moving to a tabletop. To review Chapter 3's discussion, your lower body is held on the tabletop by a spotter, while you extend your upper torso out over the edge so that you can bend to the floor. The hands can be held at the head, or the arms may be crossed on the chest. From this starting position (upper torso at 90 degrees to the tabletop), elevate the torso to horizontal (parallel to the floor). Begin by lifting at the head, but keep the back *straight* as you rise. *Do not* go more than a few inches beyond parallel. Start with a comfortable number of repetitions and progress to 40. You may hold a dumbbell against your chest to increase the intensity of the exercise. Start light (perhaps two pounds), progress to 40 reps, then increase the weight slightly.

6

BYE-BYE BODY FAT

You won't find many exercise scientists more convinced than I that strength training machines are the safest and quickest way to change the shape of the body. The intensity they allow literally forces the body to adapt by growing and improving. However, the burning of body fat off the abdominals through focused exercise of those muscles just ain't so!

As I noted earlier, spot reduction has been the huckster's promise of the ages but has been shown to be impossible. Each human body is programmed to draw body fat from specific sites in a specific order. Exercising the muscles of the outer thigh will not necessarily cause the body to release fat-mobilizing hormone (a real substance), send it to the outer thigh, then burn the released and liquified fat for energy. Would that it were true! And, of course, the same bad news is true for the abdominals: Working them in any manner will not necessarily cause the local breakdown of body fat.

Earlier, I referred briefly to my good friend and mentor Dr. Frank Katch, who is chairman of the Department of Exercise Science at the University of Massachusetts at Amherst. Frank, with his brother Victor (holding seats in both pediatric cardiology and exercise physiology at the University of Michigan), and Dr. Bill McArdle, head of the Queens College Applied Physiology Lab in New York City, have made major contributions to the understanding of metabolism, weight control, and exercise. Frank and his graduate students have completed and published two studies in the past year that drive home the truth: There is no spot reduction.

The modus operandi in both studies was to exercise a muscle or muscle group, then analyze the changes in thickness of the body fat deposit above the muscle. Let me note first that the abdomen in particular can be viewed as having three distinct layers: skin on the outer surface; a layer of subcutaneous, or below-the-skin body fat; then a deeper layer of abdominal musculature. Using newly developed X-ray techniques, Katch and his group demonstrated that literally thousands of abdominal and forearm contractions had no effect on the thickness of subcutaneous fat, though they had major effects on the underlying muscle. That is, exercise trained, strengthened, and firmed the underlying layer of muscle, but did not cause the body to burn the fat lying just above that muscle. Here's a schematic of what happened through exercise:

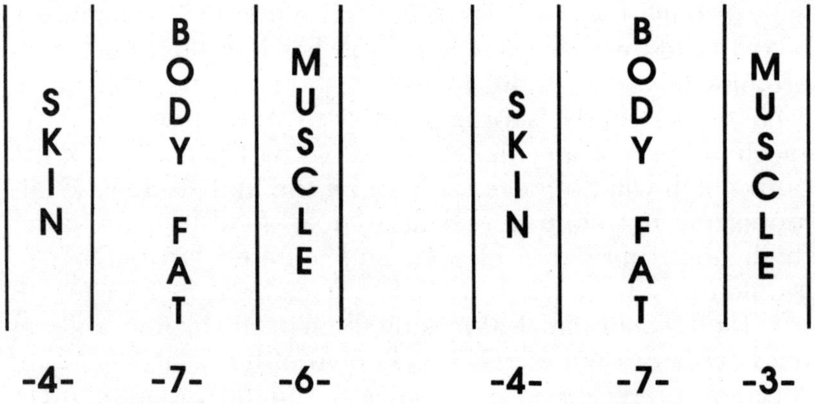

SKIN	BODY FAT	MUSCLE
-4-	-7-	-6-

Before Exercise

SKIN	BODY FAT	MUSCLE
-4-	-7-	-3-

After Exercise

On the left, the thickness of the three layers is denoted by the arbitrary numbers *4, 7,* and 6. After exercise, note that the thickness of the skin and fat layers was unchanged, while the muscle layer halved in size. The net result: the total size decreased from 17 to 14.

What does this look like on your body? With clothes on, you look slimmer and trimmer, your silhouette shrinking as the abdominal muscles tighten and draw the *unchanged* fat and skin layers inward. No one else will know you're carrying just as much fat as before—until you take your clothes off.

So how *does* one get rid of body fat? Until just about a year ago, scientists thought that it was merely a case of burning up more calories than you take in. (In fact, most of what you *still* read and hear hasn't caught up with the state of knowledge. You may be hearing the "calories out greater than calories in" line for some time.) It turns out that there's more to burning body fat than creating a negative calorie balance (out greater than in).

Of course, I'm not suggesting that the idea has been totally discarded. There *is* a rough relationship. No amount of exercise (at least no amount you're likely to perform more than once!) will lead to weight loss if you eat 7,500 calories a day. But to understand weight control and what you can do about it, you really need to go deeper. I'll keep you in shallow water here, but recommend you explore the writings of Dr. Martin Katahn for the whole story. (*The 200-Calorie Solution* and *Beyond Diet* are his two bestsellers.)

YOUR BASELINE METABOLISM—BMR

Your body has a physiological idling speed—the energy it burns while at total rest. The number of calories burned in a totally inactive state is called the *basal metabolic rate,* or *BMR.* It ranges in normal, healthy adults from as low as 1,000 for smaller women to as high as 2,500 in large males.

To obtain a picture of just how many calories one burns in a day, the sum of calories expended in work and leisure activities must be added to the BMR. An inactive, small woman may check in at 1,400 or fewer total calories expended, while a lumberjack may reach 7,000 or more in a 24-hour period.

Again, there is a rough correspondence between how much you burn and how much you eat. A lumberjack burning 7,000 calories a day will definitely lose body weight on a 3,000-calorie intake. But we're not talking about lumberjacks. We're talking about women and men who seem to eat less and less yet *not* lose weight. We're talking about fad diets that offer you 700 calories a day, which leave you hungry and eventually fatter than you were before. What's the deal?

BODY WISDOM

Your body is no dummy. It doesn't capriciously choose a random number for a basal metabolic rate. "Oh, let's burn, say, 1,250 calories today. Wonder how that sounds?" Your BMR is a direct function of your own unique chemistry. It reflects the running condition of your engines. If they're running at full speed, your BMR will be high. If you spend your waking hours sitting on the train, sitting at your desk, sitting at lunch and dinner, and sitting in front of the TV, your BMR will show it clearly. But as you change your activity patterns, BMR responds. It's why you put on that extra weight in the first place. Who among us ever sat this much back in the old high school or college days? The combination of activity and high BMR let us get away with nutritional murder. How I long for my swim team days of whole pizzas, quarts of nondiet soda, and the ice cream chaser!

But the real world caught up with you and all of us, and you slowed down and got serious—more responsibility, more money, less leisure time for calorie-burning pursuits. And as your activity level decreased, your internal chemistry slowed right along with it. There was less and less of a reason for your engines to be running at high speed, so your BMR dropped right along with the energy you expended in physical activities. But did your eating habits change? Of course not. That's what all that extra money you were earning was being spent on!

At some point you got wise to it, cut out bread (bad move; more on that later) and desserts (better move), and cut your caloric expenditure by 500 calories a day. Someone in your favorite magazine or the Sunday paper told you that 3,500 calories equaled one pound of fat and that, if you cut back 500 calories a day for seven days and burned up as many as before, you'd lose one pound a week. As far back as mathematics class was, you still could multiply seven times 500, so what could go wrong?

Well, something did. You did lose weight on your bathroom scale. In fact, it seemed just to melt away at first. Then it stopped. And you were starving but maintaining your weight. Boredom, depression, and dissatisfaction set in, and you waved bye-bye to the diet. A truly amazing thing then happened. You resumed your normal eating pattern, consuming the same number of calories as you had prediet. You had been stable at that amount, neither gaining nor losing weight. So why was that same number of calories now slapping fat onto your frame? You and millions of other dieters experienced the BMR-slowdown phenomenon. You were eating just what you ate before, but now it was making you fat.

Here's what the last two years of metabolic research have taught us: Your BMR "sensed" that you had cut your intake from 2,300 calories a day to 1,800. It didn't like it one bit. It had a body to run—cells to maintain and grow, thinking, breathing, speaking, laughing, and a few other activities that all require energy. It had only one choice when you took away 500 of its precious calories: It slowed you, and thereby itself, down. By repairing itself and growing new tissue at a slower-than-normal rate, the body could save calories. Mental and physical laziness could conserve even more. In as little as a week's time, BMR started to meet the challenge you gave it. In several weeks' time, your BMR dropped by 500 calories.

And high school math failed. Seven times 500 did indeed equal 3,500 calories. You *were* burning 3,500 less a week. But *your BMR had also dropped by 500 calories a day,* and seven times 500 equals 3,500 here, too. You were burning 3,500 less, eating 3,500 less, and your wonderful fad diet no longer worked.

So, back to the old diet of 2,300 calories a day. But look what was happening now: Your BMR was set at 1,800, *not* 2,300. Your old, comfortable daily intake was now 500 calories *greater* than your expenditure. Seven times 500 equals 3,500, and you were gaining a pound of fat a week. What a nasty trick!

THE BAD NEWS IS THE GOOD NEWS

While the adaptability of BMR to your caloric intake (as well as the drop in calories expended in physical activity) was what helped get you in trouble in the first place, it is at the same time part of the solution to the body fat problem. Your BMR does not have to drop when you begin to eat calorie-smart. What's more, BMR will *increase* as you add aerobic exercise to your lifestyle again. The more active you are, the higher it gets. By eating and exercising wisely, you can take complete control of your physiological fate and break the body fat problem.

BODY FAT SOLUTION 1: THE SWITCH TO SMART EATING

The first part of the two-pronged attack is a makeover of what and how you eat. We'll start there. Part two is the use of aerobic exercise to accomplish dual goals: an increase in calories expended through activity *plus* an increase in BMR.

What is the net result of all this work, besides improved health and resistance to disease? Body fat will disappear as you (1) rev your BMR to burn extra calories around the clock, (2) burn more calories through additional exercise, and (3) become more efficient at burning the nutrients you consume. (Author Covert Bailey coined the term *better butter burner* to describe how people become more effective users of what they eat, especially fats.)

It's as much when you eat as what you eat. One of the other problems in the "seven times 500" equation is that the timing and sizes of your meals play a critical role in body fat creation or reduction. Four meals of 700 calories each will have a totally different effect on the system than one 2,800-calorie feast. I call it the "bathtub analogy."

Picture a tub with a drain that will let out one gallon of water per minute. You may fill the tub at any rate you like, but when you get to the top, adding anything more than one gallon per minute will cause the tub to overflow. The body can be considered to have its own one-gallon-per-minute drain—it can break down and process only so much food at any one time. Anything greater will overflow and be first converted to, then stored as, body fat.

The significance of this physiological fact is that your "skip breakfast–no time for lunch–massive dinner" days must end if you want to solve the body fat problem. I wasn't kidding when I spoke of four 700-calorie meals before—that's the optimal way to consume 2,800 calories. Think of your metabolic drain as being able to handle a 700-calorie flow. Anything greater finds its way into fat cells. Is four 700s better than three 933s? Yes. Is it always practical? Unfortunately, no. What I do, and recommend, is to spread my daily calories out as much as possible. As a result, I am rarely hungry (well, rarely ravenously hungry), and I don't have to face the 2,800-calorie dinner problem.

Eat early and bigger. We've also discovered recently that body fat can be beaten by eating your larger meals earlier in the day. Apparently, the higher-calorie burn during the active daylight hours makes a greater draw on the foods you eat. Larger meals consumed later in the day appear to suffer a different metabolic fate, finding their way to fat storage more quickly. In simple terms, metabolized foodstuffs that aren't immediately used for energy (which might happen earlier in the day) find their way more quickly to storage as fat at night. Mom was right on target when she told you to eat a big breakfast.

SUMMARY EATING ADVICE:
Eat smaller meals, and more of them, at earlier times in the day.

The Columbia University Plan

I've made it easy for you: The plan that follows is a simple yet brilliant solution to the difficulties of choosing the right foods, from the right food groups, in the right amounts. It was created by nutritional scientists at Columbia University's College of Physicians and Surgeons and requires only that you select the total number of calories you want to consume. You then refer to the Daily Portion Guide and follow the bouncing ball.

How do you determine which of the four calorie-level plans—1,000, 1,200, 1,500, and 1,800—you should work with? It *will* take a little analysis. You should obtain a guide to caloric content of food and analyze several typical days' worth of food intake. Choose the Columbia University plan that comes closest to what you are eating now. Be aware that, as your BMR starts climbing from the increase in aerobic activity, you'll be able to jump up to the next-higher calorie plan. With the habits you develop from use of the plan, you'll be able to adapt to calorie intakes above 1,800.

Where are the desserts and other goodies? The fact that they're not there doesn't mean you can never eat them again. The hope is that you'll choose them a bit less frequently and adjust your caloric intake from the chart accordingly. I've got the value of a bag of M&Ms memorized: 240 calories. If I do slip and have a bag, 240 calories will have to disappear somewhere else.

Finally, since transport and storage time of fresh foods, and many of our favorite methods of food preparation, take such a toll on the nutrient values of what we eat, I do recommend a multivitamin-plus-mineral supplement. There is still little widely accepted research that megadoses of vitamins or minerals are worth their enormous expense.

FOOD EXCHANGES

List 1—Free foods
(no specific amounts)

- Bouillon
- Chicory
- Chinese cabbage
- Clear broth
- Coffee
- Endive
- Escarole
- Gelatin, unsweetened
- Lemon
- Lettuce (all kinds)
- Lime
- Mustard
- Parsley
- Pickle, sour or unsweetened dill
- Radishes
- Tea
- Soy sauce
- Vinegar
- Watercress

List 2—Vegetables
(½ cup cooked or 1 cup raw, except as indicated)

- All leafy greens, except those in List 1
- Asparagus
- Bean sprouts
- Beans, green or wax
- Beets
- Broccoli
- Brussels sprouts
- Cabbage (all kinds)
- Carrots
- Catsup (2 tablespoons)
- Cauliflower
- Celery
- Cucumbers
- Eggplant
- Mushrooms
- Okra
- Onions
- Peppers, red or green
- Rutabaga
- Sauerkraut
- Summer squash
- Tomato or vegetable juice (6 ounces)
- Tomatoes

List 3—Fruits

Apple, ½ medium
Applesauce, ½ cup
Apricots, dried, 4 halves
Apricots, fresh, 2 medium
Bananas, ½ small
Blueberries, ½ cup
Grapes, 12
Honeydew, ⅓ medium
Mango, ½ small
Nectarine, 1 small
Orange, 1 small
Papaya, ⅓ medium
Peach, 1 medium
Pear, 1 small
Pineapple, ½ cup
Cantaloupe, ¼ medium
Cherries, 10 large
Dates, 2
Figs, dried, 1 small
Fruit cocktail, canned, ½ cup
Grapefruit, ½ small
Prunes, dried, 2
Raisins, 2 tablespoons
Strawberries, ¾ cup
Tangerine, 1 large
Watermelon, 1 cup cubed
Juices:
  Grapefruit, Orange, ½ cup
  Apple, Pineapple, ⅓ cup
  Grape, Prune, ¼ cup

List 4—Starches

Breads

Any loaf, 1 slice
Bagel, ½
Dinner roll, 1, 2-inch diameter
English muffin, ½
Bun (hamburger or hot dog), ½ inch
Cornbread, 1½-inch cube
Tortilla, 1, 6-inch diameter

Cereals

Hot cereal, ½ cup
Dry flakes, ⅔ cup
Dry puffed, 1½ cups
Bran, 5 tablespoons
Wheat germ, 2 tablespoons
Pasta, ½ cup
Rice, ½ cup

Desserts

Fat-free sherbet, ½ cup
Angel food cake, 1½-inch square

Vegetables

Beans or peas (dried), ½ cup cooked
Corn, ⅓ cup (½ ear)
Parsnips, ⅔ cup
Potato, white, 1 small or ½ cup
Pumpkin, ¾ cup
Winter squash, ½ cup

Crackers

Graham, 2, 2½-inch
Matzoh, ½, 4 inches x 6 inches
Melba toast, 4
Oyster, 20
Pretzels, 8 rings
RyKrisps, 3
Saltines, 5

Alcohol

Beer, 5 ounces
Whiskey, 1 ounce
Wine, dry, 2½ ounces
Wine, sweet, 1½ ounces

List 5—Proteins

Beef, dried, chipped, 1 ounce
Beef, lamb, pork, veal, lean only 1 ounce
Lobster, 1 small tail
Oysters, clams, shrimp, 5 medium
Tuna (in water), ¼ cup
Salmon, pink, canned, ¼ cup
Cottage cheese, uncreamed, ¼ cup
Poultry, no skin, 1 ounce
Fish, 1 ounce
Egg, 1 medium
Hard cheese, ½ ounce
Peanut butter, 2 teaspoons

List 6—Milk

Buttermilk, fat-free, 1 cup
Yogurt, plain, made with nonfat milk, ¾ cup
Skim milk, 1 cup
1-percent-fat milk, 7 ounces

List 7—Fats

Avocado, ⅛, 4-inch diameter
Bacon, crisp, 1 slice
Butter, margarine, 1 teaspoon
French dressing, 1 tablespoon
Mayonnaise, 1 teaspoon
Oil, 1 teaspoon
Olives, 5 small
Peanuts, 10
Roquefort dressing, 2 teaspoons
Thousand Island dressing, 2 teaspoons
Walnut, 6 small

DAILY PORTION GUIDE: NUMBER OF PORTIONS FOR VARIOUS CALORIE LEVELS

	Calories			
List	**1,000**	**1,200**	**1,500**	**1,800**
1—Free Foods	Unlimited	Unlimited	Unlimited	Unlimited
2—Vegetables	2	2	2	2
3—Fruits	3	3	3	3
4—Starches	3	5	7	9
5—Proteins	6	6	7	7
6—Milk	2	2	2	3
7—Fats	2	2	6	7

SAMPLE MENU FOR 1,500-CALORIE PLAN

List	Number of Portions	Possible Food Choices
		MORNING
3	1	½ grapefruit
4	2	1 slice whole wheat bread and 1½ cups puffed cereal
7	1	1 teaspoon margarine
6	1	1 cup skim milk
1	—	Coffee
		NOON
5	2	½ cup tuna
4	2	2 slices bread
7	3	2 teaspoons mayonnaise and 1 teaspoon oil
2	1	3 slices tomato
3	1	½ cup diced pineapple
1	—	Lettuce, pickles, lemon juice, vinegar
		EVENING
2	1	½ cup string beans
5	4	4 ounces chicken (no skin)
4	2	½ cup mashed potatoes and ½ cup sherbet
7	2	2 teaspoons margarine
3	1	2 dates
1	—	Lettuce, radishes, soy sauce, parsley
		SNACK
6	1	1 cup skim milk
4	1	1½-inch square angel food cake
1	—	Coffee

Source: Nutrition and Health *1, 2 (1979), Columbia University Institute of Human Nutrition.*

BODY FAT SOLUTION 2: AEROBIC EXERCISE

While smart eating is absolutely essential to the body fat breakdown plan, it's aerobic exercise that will really turn the trick. Again, it accomplishes the magic through two effects: calories that are burned directly through activity and extra calories that are burned around the clock through the elevation of basal metabolic rate. In fact, this latter benefit of aerobic exercise turns out to fulfill one of mankind's oldest and fondest wishes—a means to burn calories while sitting still.

The elevation of BMR through aerobic exercise is a recently discovered phenomenon. While we are still learning the details, we know several things for certain. Most importantly, the elevation in BMR becomes a relatively fixed or permanent phenomenon. Adding three or four 20-minute aerobic bouts to your week appears to be all that's necessary to cause a significant and fat-burning rise in BMR. Think what a 200-calorie-per-day boost means over the course of one year: 200 times 365 translates to 73,000 calories, or the equivalent of 20+ pounds of fat!

The boost in BMR from aerobic exercise also has a transient, or shorter, component. In the four to eight hours after you work out, your body is still spinning along metabolically. One study presented at the 1984 meeting of the American College of Sports Medicine showed that BMR was up about 50 calories per hour over normal at the four-hour–postexercise point and actually got higher, instead of slowing down, in the hours that followed. Let me reiterate for those of you who missed that point: The people who exercised aerobically sat around and did nothing for eight hours afterward, yet burned 50–70 calories more per hour than usual. That's an offer no one can refuse.

Why Does the Exercise Have to Be Aerobic in Nature?

There's the key question. Why can't you just use your Nautilus workout to fill the exercise quota? Because only truly aerobic exercise forces the body to break down and burn fat for energy. Unless the criteria that I'll lay out in the pages ahead are met exactly, your exercise can keep your heart rate at 200 beats per minute for half an hour, but it won't be aerobic. The national misconception over just what aerobic exercise is has been the toughest nut for me (and my colleagues) to crack.

Just as I begged off the long dissertations earlier, I'll do it again now. What matters here is that you understand that heart rate is only one of the criteria that must be met for exercise to be considered aerobic. If you keep your heart rate in your training zone (more on this later), but fail to follow the other rules, you will not glean the body fat benefits of aerobic exercise.

The Rules of the Road

For exercise to be aerobic; cause a "training effect" in the heart, circulatory system, and muscles; and have the above-noted effects on basal metabolic rate and body fat, these rules must be followed:

- The heart rate must remain in or near the target zone for at least 12 minutes.
- The exercise must use one or more of the largest muscle groups in the body (quadriceps/front thigh, hamstrings/rear thigh, gluteus/buttocks, or latissimus dorsi/mid-back).
- The exercise must use those muscles rhythmically or continuously.

Perhaps an example or 11 would help. All the following meet the second and third criteria; performing them in the target heart rate zone gives you truly aerobic exercise.

- running/jogging
- swimming
- bicycling
- rowing
- cross-country skiing
- aerobic dancing (but only if well choreographed)
- stair climbing
- rope jumping

- ice or roller skating
- minitrampolines (rebounders)
- super-circuit training (combining truly aerobic stations and strength stations)

So much for your choices. Here's how you go about structuring an aerobic workout.

The Prescription for Aerobic Exercise

1. Intensity

The first of three variables you must plan is the intensity of exercise. As noted above, your heart rate—the best measure of intensity—must be in a target zone for maximal aerobic benefits. The famous formula for computing this target zone is 220 minus AGE times .70. This gives you the target number, which gets lower as you age. (Your maximal heart rate, estimated at 220 minus your age, declines as you age.) There's a better formula, though, which takes into account your resting heart rate (RHR). Since two individuals of the same age might have resting pulses (an excellent sign of fitness) that are 50 beats apart, it makes little sense to use the 220-minus-your-age formula. If my resting pulse is 40, and yours is 80, we won't have the same target heart rate. I prefer the Karvonen formula:

$$[(220 - \text{AGE} - \text{RESTING HEART RATE}) \times .70] + \text{RHR}$$

Example: AGE = 30   RESTING HEART RATE = 75

$$\begin{aligned} \text{TARGET HEART RATE} &= [\ ((220 - 30 - 75) \times 0.7) + 75\ ] \\ &= [(115 \times .07) + 75\ ] \\ &= [80.5 + 75\ ] \\ &= 155.5 \text{ BEATS PER MINUTE} \end{aligned}$$

The target zone is computed by adding and subtracting 10 beats to the target number. In this example, the target zone would be 145–165 beats per minute.

You may take your pulse at the carotid artery (along the windpipe) or along the radial artery on the thumb side of the wrist. Ten or 15 seconds is a sufficient interval; multiply by six or four to get the pulse in beats per minute.

2. Duration

Just how long must the pulse be kept in the target zone? After a warm-up of at least five minutes—preferably the activity you're about to perform but at a very low intensity—you'll need to keep the pulse in or near the target zone for at least 12 minutes. Is 20 better? Yes. Is 30 better than 20? Yes. If what you're after is fat breakdown, your goal is increased duration at a lower intensity. You might want to stick to the lower side of the target zone so you can last 40 or more minutes. If all you're after is aerobic fitness, 30 minutes is all anybody not in competition needs. And don't forget to bring yourself down slowly with an easy cool-down of at least five minutes. It's good for the heart, helps clean the waste products out of muscle, and may reduce next-day soreness.

The secret to long-duration aerobics for the out-of-shape: interval training. Many of you just had a good laugh at my 40-minute suggestion, since you'd be happy to make five minutes on the stationary bike sitting in your bedroom. The answer to all your troubles is interval training.

All you're going to do is exercise a little, then rest a little. We'll make it formal and call it the alternation of work bouts and rest intervals, but it's the same thing. Since you are sneaking in those little rest breaks, you become capable of lasting far longer. Rank beginners start with lots of rest and short work intervals, then gradually decrease the rest while lengthening the exercise intervals. I start people jumping rope with eight sequences of 15 seconds of jumping followed by 45 seconds of rest. Week two lengthens the jumping to 20 seconds and shortens the rest to 40, and week three might go to 30 jumping and 30 resting. The number of these sequences also increases, so by the end of the third week, the person might be jumping 12 30-30 sequences.

The big news: you are receiving aerobic benefits during the rest intervals! You lose nothing when compared to performing a continuous 12-minute bout of exercise. I recommend that anyone having difficulty in increasing the duration of aerobic exercise give interval training a try. (More details on writing an interval training prescription, or ITP, are found in *The Complete Book of Nautilus Training*, Contemporary Books, 1984.)

3. Frequency

As I put it in my first book, "How many times do you have to go through this each week?" The minimum frequency for training gains and body fat/BMR effects is three a week, preferably spread out over the course of the seven days. The upper limit—i.e., the maximum number of workouts—depends on how intense the workouts are. If you are working so hard that your body needs the 48 hours of rest, six aerobic workouts a week are out of the question. If your aerobics take the form of 20-minute stationary bike rides, or three-mile runs, five or six workouts a week are probably tolerable. Listen to your body. It will tell you if you are overworking. Fatigue and lingering aches and pains are the best signs.

SUMMARY

I never said it was going to be easy. All the details are here in this chapter for you to begin a concerted effort to eat smart and exercise smart. Tie these in with your torso training and you'll be a sight to see in no time flat.

7 THE TOTAL TORSO PROGRAM

Enough of the incidentals—let's get to the program!

What follows is the comprehensive plan for strengthening the lower back and trimming the middle, utilizing:

- stretching and warm-up moves to prepare properly;
- either *both* Nautilus home machines or one of the two (if you've bought only one);
- safe and supereffective calisthenics to supplement the machines;
- aerobic exercise; and
- smart eating (to complete the two-pronged attack on body fat).

This program was *not* handed to me on stone tablets. In fact, there is no exercise program on earth that was so delivered. What you read here is my best educated guess as to what will rid you of body fat, strengthen and hopefully injury-proof your back, and ripple your stomach. It will not work exactly the same for everyone. *You* are responsible for modifying and adapting it to your body and your needs.

I have intentionally started you at the lowest intensities

possible, since so many of you do not presently feature rippling abs and cast-iron backs. Some of you will move quickly to higher resistances; others will progress at a slower rate. Some will like the calisthenics; some won't. What counts is that you tune in to your body and listen to what it tells you. Pain, for example, can be either good or bad, depending on its location. Listen to it. A burning sensation in the middle of a muscle is OK; a sharp pain in a joint is not. Almost *any* pain in the back is not, especially if any tingling or numbness sensations accompany it in the buttocks or legs. Pay attention and don't work through a pain on the premise that it will go away if you ignore it. If you feel persistent pain, you should consult a physician.

The three Total Torso Programs (TTP) presented on pages 70–72 are designed for the equipment you have:

- for owners of both Nautilus Home Machines
- for owners of the Back Machine
- for owners of the Abdominal Machine

I recommend giving your complete program a serious try (a minimum of three weeks) before making modifications.

THE PROGRAM

Monday-Wednesday-Friday

Knees to Chest Modified Plow Torso Twist	Hold 20 seconds, repeat 2–3 times.
Back Machine	**Warm-up set** of 20 reps, no resistance. **Training set** at desired level of resistance, momentary muscular failure to be reached at about the 40th rep.

Tuesday-Thursday-Saturday

Abdominal Machine	Training set at desired level of resistance, momentary muscular failure to be reached at about the 40th rep.
Aerobic Exercise	Following guidelines in Chapter 6, aim for a minimum time in heart rate target zone of 12 minutes.

NOTE: Aerobic exercise is scheduled for Tuesday-Thursday-Saturday to allow the stressed lower back to recover and rebuild properly from its M-W-F training. If your back work is performed in the morning, you may try aerobic exercise later on the same day, but be on the lookout for back weakness or pain.

THE PROGRAM

Monday-Wednesday-Friday

Knees to Chest Modified Plow Torso Twist	Hold 20 seconds, repeat 2–3 times.
Back Machine	**Warm-up** set of 20 reps of no resistance. **Training set** at desired resistance, momentary failure to be reached at about the 40th rep.

Tuesday-Thursday-Saturday

Basic Curl-Up	Build to 50 reps.
Leg Exchange	Build to 100 reps, then progress to Leg Exchange with Torso Twist, building to 100 reps.
Side Leg Throws	Build to 30 reps, then progress to Assisted Leg Throws, building again to 30 reps.
Aerobic Exercise	Follow instructions in Chapter 6. Aim for a minimum time in target heart rate zone of 12 minutes.

NOTE: Aerobic exercise is scheduled for Tuesday-Thursday-Saturday to allow the lower-back musculature time to repair and rebuild after its Monday-Wednesday-Friday work. Should you train your back in the morning, you may attempt aerobic training later on the same day, provided you are wary of back pain or fatigue.

THE PROGRAM

Monday-Wednesday-Friday

Knees to Chest Modified Plow Torso Twist	Hold 20 seconds, repeat 2–3 times.
Back Extensions	Begin on floor, progressing to 40 reps. Advanced version is off tabletop with a spotter; progress to 40 reps.

Tuesday-Thursday-Saturday

Abdominal Machine	Training set with desired level of resistance. Aim for momentary failure at about the 40th rep.
Aerobic Exercise	Follow guidelines in Chapter 6. Aim for a minimum of 12 minutes in the target heart rate zone.

NOTE: Your Back Extensions will not be as stressful as work on the Back Machine, so you should have less difficulty in performing aerobically on Mondays, Wednesdays, and Fridays, if you so choose.

THE TOTAL TORSO PROGRAM FOR OWNERS OF BOTH MACHINES

You'll use your machines only three times a week, but for safety and optimal results, I'm recommending an alternate-days scheme. (I'm seeing too much low-back stress from Abdominal Machine use to suggest that they be used on the same day.)

Too much stress *cannot* be put on the value of stretching *every day* for low-back health and integrity. The three back stretches in your TTP should be done at least five days per week. A more complete stretching program is presented in *The Better Back Book* (Michael Wolf Ph.D. and Julie Davis, Contemporary Books, 1984).

I've left out exact times of day for the TTP components for one important reason: Everyone has unique body rhythms that dictate when peak physical performance is most likely. You may already be tuned into your "chronobiology," knowing the times of day you are "up" and energy-charged and those when you would kill for a quiet little nap. Here again I'll leave it up to you; analyze your physical performance on the stretches, calisthenics, and machines. Even those of you (like me) who are wide awake and raring to go at 6:00 A.M. may find that the muscles of the back need an hour or two more than you do to wake up. If you do happen to find wake-up-time training OK, give later-afternoon or evening work a shot in case the results are even better.

APPENDIX CHARTING YOUR TOTAL TORSO PROGRAM

On the following pages are charts that can be used to record your progress in stretching, machine work, calisthenics, and aerobic exercise. Each chart covers a week's worth of work, so in all, you have a 10-week program (more if you make photocopies of a blank chart).

ing of one of the buildings, extolled the stone and cedar exterior and finished with the statement:

Last but not least, Cody Place roofing is made out of impervious metal.
Your roofing is guaranteed for a lifetime of satisfaction.

Jella read this to the group and a smile crossed the face of everyone but the man with the hard hat. She completed her presentation.

"This seems to point a finger at the developer, AJA Capital that has, in effect, made a written guarantee. We must, however, be sure of what actually happened and this is why we wanted you all here today." At that, Jella nodded to Bill Berkowitz who said that he wanted to hear from the others present. The structural engineer was the first to rise.

"I don't see how there could have been any structural failures. In the first place, every roof joist and beam is designed to carry a maximum snow load. I believe I'm right that this roof was applied after last winter's snow melted so that any leaks would be from relatively light rainfall, not from heavy snow loads."

"I think that I can help with this," said the architect. "We research metal roofs before ever specifying them on any job. The best roof would be one without any seams but that's nearly impossible. Therefore, all the metal roofing manufacturers supply sheets with raised seams that are folded over where the sheets meet. With possible temperature differences of 100 degrees at that altitude, these seams move as the metal expands and they may eventually open up enough to leak. After many years, we have settled on Arliss Metal Roofing that has a unique, patented seam that moves without opening up. Arliss was specified here and, to be totally safe, we specified a product called Ice and Water Shield manufactured by W.R. Grace. A layer under the metal will keep any water from leaking into the space below.

"We were not hired on this job to see if the work in place conforms to our construction documents. The developers said that they would use the drawings as guidelines for a construction manager to take over from there."

"Does that relieve the architect of any responsibility during construction?" questioned Bill Berkowitz.

"It should; but, as you can see, that didn't keep us out of this meeting today. That being said, on this job the construction manager took our drawings and put them through a process called Value Engineering. He probably showed the owner a dozen places where costs could be saved by using alternate materials. The basic problem is that construction managers are just consultants to the process and have no liability for errors or omissions. They can come up with plenty of

cost cuts but don't necessarily describe the deficiencies that go with the savings." Bill Berkowitz nodded his head in understanding and then turned to look at the man with the hard hat, saying,

"I assume that you represent someone in this process. Perhaps the construction managers?"

"Yes, I mean no. I should explain. My name is Sid Lowry and I was hired by AJA as a foreman for the construction. I take my orders from AJ himself, but he was only on the job three times. He told me in the beginning that this would be his baby, because he wanted to break into multi-family housing and this would be a good trial. Besides, it would be right on his way to his second home in Keystone."

"So, where does this lead us?" Jella questioned.

"Well, AJ got involved with all the work in South America and was never around to make decisions."

"What about the construction manager?"

"Oh, he was only hired to review the drawings for Value Engineering. AJ certainly didn't want any help from anybody."

"Do you recall the brand name for the roofing?" I interrupted.

"Absolutely, I recall a semi unloading all that metal, because he was blocking my access in order to make the delivery. The labels on the stuff he was delivering all said Permaroof." The architect leapt to his feet.

"That stuff is like tinfoil! There are product liability lawsuits throughout the west against the maker." Bill looked around the table and then looked back at one of the product reps. "This was your product?"

"Hell, no. I'm from Arliss and this whole thing's beginning to annoy me. Why am I here?"

"We are sorry to put you out," said Jella," but your company was named on the construction documents and we had no other information. At least you're out of the picture! Now, what about the waterproofing?" The roofer put both hands on the edge of the conference table as if he was going to push away, but thought better of the idea before answering Jella.

"We did all the roofing, just as it should have been done. We have a reputation to uphold!"

"What about the waterproofing? The Ice and Water Shield?" When Jella repeated her question, the W.R. Grace rep held back the roofer from answering and interjected,

"Our product has been in use for a decade without any failures unless the roofer failed to follow our installation instructions. What was the temperature when you installed the Ice and Water Shield?"

"Ice water shield? What the hell is that? I come from Limon. All my men come from Limon. It's high desert country. We've never heard of the material, so how can you expect us to put it in?"

At that, Bill excused the structural engineer and the reps for W.R. Grace and Arliss roofing with great apologies and a suggestion that they both go below for a hearty lunch to be billed to Bates Brown & Berkowitz. He asked the roofer and Sid Lowry to wait while the plaintiffs held a brief conference. We agreed that suing the roofer was probably a waste of time and that AJA Capital was definitely the party at fault.

AJ Arneson, and AJA Capital were informed that a suit would be filed for all damages unless the developer re-built all the roofs according to the architect's specifications, re-built all the damaged ceilings, employed the architect to inspect the work and presented a check for $10,000 to each of the affected unit owners for incidental damages and suffering. All this was to be done within 45 days. The roofer was told that he was obviously part of the problem and should expect a claim from AJA that he'd have to settle.

During a hurried call to Mexico City, Swathey was told to take care of the problem because AJ didn't have time. He was tied up on a bid for a new bridge between El Paso and Ciudad Juarez. Sylvia received the required repairs and a check for $10,000 within 30 days. Along with the check was a note that said in part,

> *Although others caused the error, President A.J. Arneson of AJA Capital wants to be sure that the work has been completed satisfactorily. We look forward to sharing many happy times with you in this soon-to-be-sold-out project.*

35.

Celebration of the victory against AJ Arneson was short lived as the Willow Glen case grew closer to a resolution. On the following Wednesday, Jella and I met Bob Duer at the courthouse for the first meeting with the judge that would handle Willow Glen. Jella was dressed in her serious suit, the one that told the world that she was a dedicated attorney. She even had on a pair of horn-rimmed glasses that I knew were not prescription.

I assumed that the meeting was a prelude to a trial and was looking forward to my first chance to present evidence before jury members who would determine the guilty party. I still wasn't sure who that was, but I was proud of the work I'd done to date and the fact that justice would prevail. It was obvious that the construction process was rife with legal potholes and it was time to fill some of the holes and discourage repeats of the same errors. An end to the dispute was coming and I was hoping for another victory for our team.

We took an elevator to the meeting room floor to find a crowd of more than a dozen people. Jella shook hands with a few and I nodded towards Alex Gordano and Fernando Gonzalez. The place was filled with attorneys representing the defendants plus those in addition that worked for the liability insurance companies. The buzz around the large conference table quieted as a man in a black robe that almost hid his jeans and madras shirt, walked into the room. Jella poked me and murmured,

"Judge Pearson."

The judge sat down at the head of the table, introduced himself and then turned to a young woman seated behind a black typing box and a stack of paper.

He explained that although this was not a calendared hearing, he wanted this court recorder to take notes unless any of the participants objected. He then asked each person to identify themselves and their reasons for being there, starting with the man on his left.

"I am Cedric Smith, general manager of Transit Mix Cement Corporation. We are a branch of a national firm that supplies twenty per cent of all the cement delivered in the United States. Our products are all mined within the States and last year our total sales volume ..."

"Stop right there!" the judge ordered. "We have a lot to do here and I don't want a lot of BS sales information. Please limit your statements to the part your organization played in producing what appears to be a huge pile of rubble. I've looked at that mess in Broomville and only wish that the suit hadn't been filed in my court."

Pearson was even more blunt than the judge at Jerry Studely's hearing. It was easy to see how the law differed from the practice of architecture. While there were numerous ways to solve a design problem, there was no wiggle room with the law. Moreover, an architect presents his case to the world but a lawyer stands before one judge, and this one wasn't going to take any nonsense. Cedric Smith was a quick learner as he formed a reply.

"Yes, sir. We delivered all of the concrete for the building. All of the required tests, however, show that our product met specifications."

Next, Gonzalez described how they had cut and bent all the reinforcing bars. On Gonzalez's left was the attorney for Eldridge & Bacon accompanied by Mr. Robert Bacon. Bacon nodded but said nothing. There was a vacant chair between Bacon and David Hoyt. Hoyt explained that it was for his attorney who had been delayed in court. Hoyt then said,

"I'm the one that's been hurt by all this. I put my faith in the architects, engineers and contractors and what have I got for it? I'm losing millions on this deal before I even start."

"We all understand your position Mr. Hoyt," said the judge.

Next, a lawyer representing AJA Capital simply said that AJA was a financial partner with Mr. Hoyt who had complete responsibility fro anything that happened in the construction phase. The AJA lawyer looked for approval from a co-barrister who was there to speak for Watchtower Savings and Loan. The Watchtower rep shook his head up and down, presumably to support the implication that money, as such, was always free from any guilt.

An attorney for the company that issued professional liability insurance to the architects gave his name. He sat next to Sam Lovell of Smith & Bair. An insur-

ance agent for Dietz plus the insurer's attorney flanked Alex Gordano. A representative of UPRIGHT briefly explained his role, whereupon Judge Smith looked at Jella and asked,

"And you are?"

"I am Angela Adams, attorney for Dietz Construction and I am joined by Woodford Stickley, Architect and Robert Duer, Structural Engineer. The two gentlemen have been doing forensic research as to the cause of the building failure."

"Oh?" queried the judge. "I'd like to hear their findings."

"We will do that, Judge Smith, providing that, if there is a settlement before trial, the records of any statements here will be sealed." Jella didn't want any information that would be detrimental to Deitz to be made public if she could avoid it.

"Unusual, but acceptable unless someone here objects." I described my meetings with the various players and listed the six hypothetical reasons that could have contributed to the collapse. Bob Duer presented his test findings.

"I removed a section of the steel where it intersects the floor slabs. We tested and found that thirty percent of the welds were sub-standard. Given the factors of safety involved, thirty percent was probably not enough to have caused the collapse. I also reviewed the structural drawings and I question the location shown for reinforcing around the elevators. I did not investigate the hydraulic equipment used in lifting the slab, but there could have been failures with the so-called shearheads used to lift the slabs." The UPRIGHT rep objected.

"We have built dozens of these structures without failure. If they'd followed all our guidelines, the building would be standing today!"

"Summing up," Jella quickly said, "There are five or six areas that individually were not big problems, but in combination might have been enough to finally bring the building down." I quickly picked up from her.

"One of the major problems, here, is the fact that the developer hired the structural engineers directly, cutting out the architect's ability to coordinate the engineers in the field. The developer also contracted directly with UPRIGHT, bypassing the general contractor. The architect had no control over the engineer. Dietz had no control over UPRIGHT. Neither the contractor nor the engineers had ever used the UPRIGHT system and one might have expected UPRIGHT to offer more than the usual assistance in the field. I understand that there was confusion at each slab pour." This brought an angry look from Hoyt, who said:

"I don't know who these people are or what their qualifications may be. As far as I'm concerned they are making unfounded accusations and threaten to destroy

a development company and a reputation that I've spent years of honest hard work to establish. This is all nonsense!"

The judge nodded, looked around the table and then excused himself for a break after directing each of the parties to meet separately, consider their positions and return in one half hour. I assumed he wanted time to look at his calendar dates and review what he had to do before the trial. The Dietz defense team met in the corridor outside and tried to analyze what we'd heard. When the judge returned to his seat, we rushed to join him. As the various representatives took their seats, Judge Pearson spoke out.

"I've heard enough to believe that the complications implied here are as bad as the tangled mess of concrete and steel that I saw at the job site. A trial could keep you all in court for months, even years. You don't want that. Your insurers don't want that. The only ones that want that are the attorneys. They are always the winners.

I suggest that you submit the case to Arbitration. You will go into the process agreeing to accept the decision of the independent arbiter. He or she will listen to all of you individually and then determine an amount, if any, that each of you will be liable for due to your role in the building failure." Sam Lovell raised his hand and said,

"With your solution, we'll never know who was really at fault. How can we be sure that justice is being served?" The judge stood up and replied,

"Justice? Justice? We aren't here to determine justice. We are here to get this thing settled outside of my courtroom. I am already backlogged for six months and you may all be gone before a jury could hear the case."

Judge Pearson suggested the name of an arbitrator that was well known for handling construction cases. Everyone agreed that if he would take the case, they would participate. It took two, ten-hour days for the arbitrator to meet with each of the parties and then arrive at dollar amounts owed. When Fernando Gonzalez complained that he had nothing to do with the problem and didn't see why he should be out five thousand dollars as his share of the settlement, the arbitrator asked him if he'd rather spend a year with his attorney beside him in court.

During a break in one of our sessions, I took Al Gordano aside and asked him about the argument that I'd witnessed on my visit to AJA Capital on another case. His jaw twisted back and forth as he thought for a minute and then came up with an explanation.

"Arneson had called us in there in hopes that he could pinpoint the real cause of the collapse. He'd had his own investigators on the job and they'd arrived at conclusions similar to the ones you listed. Arneson had lost money and was look-

ing for a single entity to sue and preferably one with deep pockets. He particularly didn't want blame placed on Hoyt because he knew Hoyt was penniless. The judge outmaneuvered him."

I was unhappy that Dietz and most of the others had to pay something simply to keep them out of court; but pleased that none of the money would go to Hoyt, who claimed he was due thirty-five thousand a month for administrative services. The bulk of the money collected from all those involved went to Watchtower Savings and Loan who put up the funds in the first place.

Hoyt finally agreed to pay the largest settlement to cover his faulty management of the entire project. He would never need the money he demanded for administrative services and he would never make good on his pledge. The news came out a few months after the arbitration sessions: Hoyt was charged with criminal intent. Apparently, he was a part owner of Watchtower S&L and also a director of a similar bank in west coast Florida. He had manipulated the transfer of Watchtower's investment in Willow Glen to his Florida S&L at twice the value on Watchtower's books. He pleaded that the amounts differed because the Florida S&L was investing in developed land. Hoyt was sentenced to a year in jail for bank fraud. As I read about his sentence, my thoughts went back to one I shared with Bob and Jella when we walked out of the mediator's office.

"God, I hope we'll never see another one like this." It was only the beginning.

36.

Channel Nine TV was on so that we could catch the evening news and weather predictions for the next day. It was around nine fifty, so I'd tuned into the closing scenes of a show called Survival that was filmed on a desert island in the Pacific. According to the rules, each week the competitors had to vote out one of the members as less competent. The last to remain would win the prize money. While younger contestants were discussing ways to catch fish to survive, an older man was constructing a shelter on the beach. When the others complained that he wasn't acting like part of a team, the senior citizen shouted back.

"I'm sixty years old. When you're that old, you can give the orders, but for now I'm in charge!" The spokesman was the first to be voted out of the group. His name? AJ Arneson.

I waited patiently for any real news following the Survival program. The local channels never reported on national or international events. Jella and I had a running bet as to how many gurneys we could count each time we tuned in. I was about to turn the TV off when the newscaster introduced a special report called *Environment or Employment? Minturn Muddles over Mine.* The camera focused on a hillside scarred by what a person explained were the operations of the Ajax mine near Leadville. The voice-over said,

"Citizens in the town of Minturn are ready to fight against anything like the disaster shown here in nearby Leadville where, for years, the mighty Ajax Amalgamated has been gouging the once-sylvan mountains to extract something called molyb … molybdenum. The good news is that a little bit of molybdenum added to steel increases its strength. This means a lighter weight bicycle for all you

cyclists and possibly lighter weight cars that will reduce gas consumption. The bad news is: well, let's get some local opinions. Here's Sam Appleby. Mr. Appleby? Can I call you Sam? OK. What do you think about the new mine?" The camera panned down a block of Minturn's main street that was lined with stores. The interviewer shoved a microphone under the chin of an elderly man dressed in coveralls, a denim shirt and an S F Giants baseball cap.

"Well, Sir, I've lived here most of my life and worked at the Gilman mine since I was a teenager. That's the closed-down operation five miles up the road from here. 'Five miles and two thousand feet up. We used to drop the lead ore down the mountain to the railroad."

"But, you risked your life in that mine. Now you hear that it dumped bad chemicals into the river. Do you want more of that?"

"Do I want to see another mine? Well sir, the mine and the railroad is what's made Minturn. Since the mine closed down, Minturn's gone to hell while all the towns around us are growing because of those ski lifts. I guess opening up the mine again wouldn't hurt. Of course, we don't want any more pollution." The camera moved back to the street, broke away and moved in on a man in a wheelchair. The man was seated in front of a sign identifying the Minturn town hall. The announcer leaned over to lower the microphone to the man's face.

"Folks, I'm talking here with Mayor Melrose, who has a slightly different view. Mr. Mayor, how about a new Ajax mine just up the road from here?"

"We don't want it. Mining has ruined the mountain, ruined the river and ruined Minturn. I ran on a vow to bring back Minturn's economy, but we don't need a new mine to do that. I can't give you the details now, but talks are underway with a large recreational organization that is very close to a commitment. That's all I can say." The picture then went back to the studio where a Channel Nine spokesperson sat across a table from a man and a woman. Anchor Michael Murphy looked at the woman and introduced her as Margaret Minor, representative of a new group called SAME, Save Minturn's Environment.

"Ms. Minor, could you tell us a little about your organization? When did it start up? What are your goals? Who is supporting your effort?"

"Our goal is to preserve Minturn's special character. It is one of the oldest towns in the county and its main street contains five historic buildings built before the turn of the century. They are the IOOF Hall, Smith's Pharmacy …"

"Yes, but what about the mine?"

"We have not taken a vote yet; but we would be opposed to anything that would in any way disturb the status quo—the environmental status quo, that is. In fact right now we are partners in a lawsuit against the owners of the old mine

because they haven't followed EPA directives to clean up the river. Ajax or anybody else that comes in here will just make matters worse." Murphy turned to a man he identified as Stan Demeral from Ajax Amalgamated Mines.

"Mr. Demeral, how can you be even thinking about opening up that mine when SAME is against you, the mayor is against you and I would guess all Minturn is against you?"

"Michael, let's get some things straight here. State of the art equipment today is decades ahead of the Gilman operation. Advanced mining techniques will make it possible to extract the metal without leaving a mark on the land. Ajax Amalgamated does not intend to repeat the mistakes made with the present Gilman zinc mine. In fact, right now we are studying ways to meet the EPA directives, ways that Ajax will pay for as a prerequisite to getting the Moly from the super vein that is a mile below the present town.

"Let's talk about molybdenum ... Moly we call it. Getting to molybdenite requires hard-rock mining. Everything is done with modern machines far underground and carried to the surface on elevators. The molybdenite is crushed to get the molybdenum: no fumes, no odors, and no air pollution. And get this: Moly is vital to our national defense effort. It makes our tanks tougher, our guns lighter and is even a great lubricant."

"Thank you, Mr. Demeral. It looks like it's going to be an interesting time for Minturn. Now let's get the last word from Mayor Melrose who you can be sure is going to keep Ajax on its toes. Melrose, by the way, is a fighter that understands adversity. He says that his handicap, that we understand is the result of a combination of accidents, has inspired him to give something back to the gods for saving his life. Mr. Mayor, you have the floor."

"Thanks, Michael. The town of Minturn appreciates Channel Nine bringing the potential horrors of an Ajax mine to the attention of Colorado, and hopefully the world. Let me say this. Ajax can build its mines wherever it wants, but not in my backyard!"

Melrose's words were indicative of the kind of problems facing the state of Colorado. The state had some of the best-preserved mountain open space in the country that was ideal for outdoor recreation, but that open space also had some of the earth's more bounteous reserves of oil, gas and minerals lying under its crust. Tourist recreation, the second largest income producer in the state, depended upon the mountains; but the extractive industries wanted permits to operate in those same mountains. The question was which use was going to overwhelm the other.

Jella and I had become more aware of the conflicts. We joined the Sierra Club and donated to the Nature Conservancy. We formed a committee in our hang-gliding organization to help save the open land so necessary to our sport. As professionals we weren't sure that it was a matter of supporting one side or the other. Ski resort operators cut down as many trees as oil prospectors and both industries brought in more population that could endanger the high desert environment. We wanted to minimize environmental damage wherever it might happen. How that related to forensic investigations and construction litigation was another question.

The next day Jella called me at my office to say that Bill Berkowitz wanted to meet with the two of us. He'd suggested a lunch at the Denver Country Club, so I drove back to Jella's to change into a new blue button-down shirt, new necktie, new blue blazer and a new pair of gray flannel pants. I'll quickly confess that my bedmate was also my new sartorial mentor. If I was going to be around lawyers, I needed the right uniform.

Jella's house was only a few blocks from the tree-dotted oasis of the Denver Country Club. I parked and told the attendant at the front door that I was to meet Mr. Berkowitz. In my haste, I'd arrived fifteen minutes early so the attendant ushered me into a small waiting room. I sat in a leather chair, looked at the portraits of early Denver greats on the walls and then picked up a small leather covered book. It described how the country club was opened for golf in the early 1900's as the promotional draw for an exclusive subdivision. My Swiss chalet clients on Franklin Street were part of that subdivision. They could add the historic label to Cadillac and Saks Fifth Avenue as part of their credentials.

The book said the subdivision was supposed to be a Spanish style community because both Denver and Madrid fell near the 40th parallel. It was a geographical stretch, but a good way to sell real estate that now was the most exclusive and expensive neighborhood in Denver. The neighborhood elitism didn't seem that different from what I saw growing up in a Salt Lake City where the Temple was its own sort of club. I closed the book as I saw Jella and Bill come to get me past the gate guard.

In the dining room, the headwaiter led the three of us to a table near a window; but Bill said that he'd prefer a less crowded area. Once seated in a small alcove, I thanked Bill for inviting me to the country club. Jella gave me one of her "What?" looks, but I pretended not to notice as I pulled at my gray flannels to save the crease. After an exchange of ubiquitous questions about each other's health, Bill looked at the two of us and said,

"I suppose you're wondering why I wanted to meet with you outside the office. Let's order first. Each of you has a menu pad. Just mark off what you'd like. I recommend the small New York if you like red meat." I didn't need to look further. Bill waited for us to mark the pads before continuing. "You may have heard that Ajax Amalgamated is proposing a new mine up in the mountains not far from Vail. You may also know that Ajax is a dirty word when it comes to mines." We both nodded, understanding his statement. He continued:

"My partner Allan Brown … have you met him, Woody? No? Well Allan is what we might call old school Denver. He knows everyone in town and this has meant a great deal to the success of Bates Brown and Berkowitz. Allan sits on many corporate boards, including Ajax Amalgamated Mines. Allan called me into his office yesterday to tell me that Ajax is looking for professionals to help them fight any opposition to their Gilman mine proposal. Allan sees this like the trial lawyer he is: what Ajax needs is in depth law research that supports unrestricted mining on government lands. There are plenty of examples, particularly in Colorado. Ajax can throw every case in the books at the unreasonable opposition in Minturn."

"So," questioned Jella, "You might have some reservations about that approach?"

"Well, yes. Attitudes are changing, particularly in this state. Permits to slash timber or screw up the land are not going to be handed out on a platter. I've talked about this many times with Stan Demeral who is Ajax's in-house counsel."

"We saw him on TV last night."

"Stan is convinced that Ajax can put in a mine without damaging the environment, but they'll have to make concessions and show that they will be responsible members of the local communities. They've already cleaned up the mess left by zinc mining at Gilman, but they'll have to do more. Much more: things like direct support of local charities, building new infrastructure, providing proper housing for their employees. Stan and I have talked about forming teams of consultants to advise them on how to get their permits, given today's realities."

"So, what does that have to do with us?" asked Jella.

"I know where Allan Brown is heading. He'll advise the board to hire a law firm that is known for taking the corporation's side and fighting a project through the courts. I want to head him off with a well-thought-out proposal for a team approach that we then can make to Ajax. It will take Stan Demeral and some higher-ups to sway the board; but it's worth the gamble. This goes way beyond normal law. I need the two of you to prepare a game plan that attacks all the problems Ajax will face and shows how to resolve them.

"I want to know about housing? What about the design of the buildings? What happens when you add thousands of workers to an existing community without proper planning: more crime, residential sprawl? You need new schools, new playgrounds, and new fire stations. All that stuff. No one's talking about a better local economy, good incomes, improved community services and, cleaned-up pollution! We have to prove that the bad effects can be kept to a minimum. I've talked enough. Think about it and get back to me tomorrow with your ideas. Now let's enjoy lunch."

"I like having a law firm head up the team," I commented before cutting into my steak. "A board like Ajax will be suspicious of people like land planners, real estate developers and ex-government employees. You'll need those kinds that know their field; but they can't be looked at as tree-huggers by the board." We ate, but before we left the table Jella said,

"Woody and I talked about this after listening to that TV program. It's no secret to you that I'd like to be doing more environmental work. I've tried to avoid bugging you about that, but I know that I could contribute more to the real world than I'm doing right now. Working with the potential despoilers could be just as effective as sitting on the other side. We'll get right on it."

37.

Bill Berkowitz's idea of adequate timing was to compress a week's work into one evening. We might have had the benefit of sharing the same dinner table and the same sleeping bed, but that night there was little of either. In preparing a proposal for Bill we assumed an adversarial position against Ajax to see what we'd have to combat. I made some notes as we talked over the possible areas of concern.

- Public Relations: bad vibes
- Corporate Control: fear of Ajax domination
- Environmental Pollution: air, soil, water.
- Visual Pollution: structures and tailing piles.
- Temporary Housing: construction workers
- Employee Issues: locals vs. new, ethnic issues
- Community Impacts: crime, sprawl, infrastructure, traffic.

There were two major areas of concern: environmental damages resulting from the plant construction and community damages that might spread across the entire county. A team was needed that could identify the problems, propose mitigations and be able to sell it all to both Ajax and the general public. First,

someone had to make an environmental assessment of existing flora and fauna. We'd also need a tally of existing roads, housing, infrastructure and community services. Ajax would have to hire specialists to analyze and advise in each of these areas:

- Environmental
- Site Planning
- Building Design
- Economics
- Crime Prevention
- Housing, Urban Design
- Community Services
- Local Government
- State, Federal Government
- Public Relations

Ajax would have to start correcting impacts from the existing mine: abandoned buildings, deserted housing and land desecration. Any new construction would have to have minimal impacts, both physical and visual. Jella brought up a major problem.

"I'm sure that no one will accept a company town. Sociologists frown on places like Pullman, Indiana and Hershey, Pennsylvania. All those old houses in Gilman will have to be converted into on-site uses or torn down. This will push housing somewhere else. Without controls, the demand will create sprawl in neighboring communities. The logical place for Ajax to build housing for its workers is Minturn. That's going to take a lot of real investment beyond the mine costs."

"That's also going to take a lot of selling," I said. "First, we have Allan Brown and probably Bates, neither of whom would want to lose a good client. Then there's Mayor Melrose and the rest of the town of Minturn. Then there's the entire county that is more interested in tourism than industry. How about all the

agencies in the state and federal governments? The only two people that might be in favor of our proposal, at least we hope, are Bill and Stan Demeral from Ajax."

We put together arguments that the two of them could use to soften the contents of what would be a very debatable proposal. Hard rock miners considered themselves tough, and they carried their risk-taking arrogance whenever they left the mines for the outside world. This attitude extended from the lowest cat operator to most of the administrative staff. They were not in the habit of making concessions. It wouldn't be easy. The next day we briefed Bill on the direction that might be taken.

On Friday the three of us had our first meeting with Stan Demeral at Ajax headquarters in a new low-rise building in West Denver. All their offices opened to a central atrium space with a large glass skylight overhead. We took the elevator to the third floor and met Stan who described his position as house counsel and company janitor to clean up the mess at the Ajax mine in Leadville.

He said that at first he'd approached Leadville as a legal joust, a game where Ajax provided minimum responses to EPA demands. Each day that he went to the mine, however, brought him closer to the public attitude that Ajax had created an environmental disaster. Stan talked with the miners, sparred with Leadville politicians and listened to locals over beer at the Golden Spike. He found that people were proud of their work in the mine, proud of their community it supported, and typically in fear of the corporation that made it all possible

"Exploitation isn't a popular sport anymore," he told us. "If a corporation is going to take something out of the environment, it's got to give back in kind, even if the taking is a mile underground. At a going price of twenty-five dollars a pound, yes a pound, there should be plenty of profits to spend on employee and community relations. That's my feeling, and each day I make a little more headway with the CEO and hopefully some of it will rub off on the board. What have you three got that will help me?" Bill gave an overview of our approach.

"There are two questions about your mine: What will it do to the environment and what will it do to the community? Ajax must start by cleaning up any pollution from the existing mine. Next, Ajax will have to design a plant that fits into that hillside and makes a statement about environmental adaptation: maybe solar panels and sod roofs.

"That's not the biggest worry for the community. Where do all these new workers live? How does a town pay for all the new police, fire and educational facilities needed because of the mine? Increased traffic, crime and family quarrels! You need to hire sociologists, criminologists, economists and a good public rela-

tions expert. We've made a list." He read off my list and added a few names of his own.

"This is good," said Stan with a head nod in our direction." Everyone in Ajax knows that it's going to have to spend money to get the mine. My job will be to convince the board that it has to spend money up front to come up with answers to community concerns if it wants to get any permits at all. Then, they'll have to spend more to put the goodies in place. Let me take it from here and I'll get back to you." There was no conversation as we headed back to York Street. Jella was obviously reviewing the meeting in her mind, but finally asked what I was thinking about

"I was just trying to understand the implications of what we've just done," which wasn't at all true. What I was really thinking about was our relationship. I'd lived with this wonderful woman. We worked together as a team without arguing over methods or materials. I marveled at this person who seemed to have an in-borne trust whether it was in soaring to 13,000 feet or freely giving herself to me. It was hard to reconcile the strength required to stay aloft with the soft, smooth body that clung close to me most evenings.

The bond went beyond the bed and carried into the simplest activities as if each of us knew what the other would do without ever mentioning it. We seemed to think the same way despite our almost opposite vocations. Maybe her left-brain and my right brain had sort of a Yin-Yang relationship that meshed at the right places.

I had some sense of guilt. Not any kind of moral questioning, but the feeling that I owed Jella something more than just my love and paying my share of the expenses. My idea of guilt may not have come from Sunday school; but it was always there, probably because it was hard to grow up in Salt Lake City without being exposed to biblical thinking. I got it in the classroom, I got it on the football field and I got it at home even though my parents had never joined the church. Perhaps Martin Luther's hold on old Gustav Stickley carried down in the family genes. Outside the home we never drank coffee or tea and certainly never touched an alcoholic beverage. Even if they were not directly prohibited by the LDS, my father was too close to the church to be seen breaking the laws of the gospel according to Joseph Smith.

None of this moral sense of right and wrong was changed when I read Darwin's *On the Origin of the Species* or *The Basic Writings of Sigmund Freud.* My beliefs carried into, in fact prompted, my marriage to Karina. I felt it was the right thing to do. In fact, it was the wrong thing to do and ending it created more wrong because I'd broken my marriage vows. What of it?

What of it? Did I have to marry Jella in order to prove my love? Where did marriage come from in the first place? I'd read that the Egyptian pharaohs first instituted the concept of marriage in order to insure heredity on the throne. The Romans? They loved laws and had one for each of three different kinds of marriage depending upon how many witnesses there were. Both the Greeks and the Romans instituted the idea of a dowry, presumably so that if a wife left the household the irate husband had something to hold onto. The one thing that seemed a common thread through history was the thought that the man was in charge. I wasn't so sure that was right.

I could see that marriage originally was a good way to keep order between humans and at the same time perpetuate Homosapiens. By dividing his subjects up into family units, a ruler only had to deal with a single head. As for contemporary marriage, had the concept outlived realities? The formal bond was certainly questionable in a modern world where a divorce was as easy as tearing up a ticket for the game. So why my guilt?"

"Jesus, watch out for that pick-up!" Jella shouted as I came close to the truck in the other lane. I was obviously not watching the road. I could sense the almost negligible gap of air between the two vehicles as I held the wheel and pointed straight ahead. Happily, the truck driver didn't waver and I slowly breathed out a sigh of thanks to whatever god was watching Speer Boulevard.

38.

Stan Demeral took our ideas to the Ajax CEO and the two of them made a presentation to the board of directors. The proposal pretty much followed our recommendations with a major exception: the team would be managed by The Institute to Resolve Conflicts, IRC, an entity within the University of Denver that specialized in conflict resolution. IRC provided a forum to resolve differences between corporations and environmental activists for timber cutting, gas exploration and coal mining. It didn't hurt that Ajax was a large contributor to the university. The director of IRC, Peter Newman agreed to head up the team.

Ajax put two major efforts in motion. They hired Keyser Engineers to begin preliminary design of the proposed mine. This would start with research at the Colorado School of Mines on possible new ways to reduce the tailings usually found with hard rock mining. Keyser would lay out the mineshaft, lifting systems and the above ground manufacturing plant. Ajax also hired IRC as a counter-group to review Keyser's plans and propose mitigation measures for their impacts on the environment and the community.

Peter Newman called his new group the Planning and Conservation Committee, PCC. The PCC held monthly meetings to deal with the many negative issues that surrounded the new mine. The subject of the first meeting was *The attributes and detriments of the existing Gilman Mine.* Newman knew what he was doing. In order to get the group close to the problem he held the first meeting, a 2-day affair, in the former office building at Gilman. This was the only building still habitable and was primarily there for the use of the watchmen that patrolled the grounds.

The names of those that sat on makeshift seats around an old conference table at the first meeting were impressive. Stan was there representing Ajax. Charlie Gordan had come up from Florida. His firm had recently devised a rehab plan that turned the scarred hillsides of an abandoned Kentucky coal mine into a championship golf course. An economist from the University of Denver named Edward Greiner had studied the economic impacts of the new gas fields on the town of Rock Springs, Wyoming. Rock Springs and Sweetwater County were appropriate examples to compare with Gilman and Eagle County because over the years there'd been a succession of different mining operations for coal, soda ash, oil shale and natural gas.

Bert Lavell, former Aspen city manager, was there to assess local government issues and propose solutions. There were two representatives from the town of Carbondale: a former police chief and a criminal psychologist. He was overweight and she had the kind of beauty that Jella could hate if I continued my discreet surveillance. I just couldn't figure out how someone like that was immersed in a sea probably filled with malcontents, rapists and hatchet murderers. Jella and I were assigned to research zoning law, urban planning and housing.

Stan Demeral greeted and thanked everyone for attending the first session, adding that he hoped everyone could commit the time and remain with the group at least through the permit stage. Peter Newman assumed his role as chairman and asked for opinions about the detriments and possible attributes of the existing Gilman mine. There was consensus that the mine stood as an example of what not to do, but on the other hand it was sitting there as a sore spot waiting to be healed.

Bert Lavell from Aspen said that if adverse impacts on the environment could be overcome, he thought that the problems related to a population boom could also be solved. He mentioned the impacts and mitigations that had been made over the years in his county and looked to the two from Carbondale in hopes they might pick up his lead. The chief, Ezra Smiley, said that the boom was bringing in new housing, new businesses and a tax base and the increase in taxes would support a proper police force and other public services. The psychologist, Martha Merritt, described the way social problems had been attacked and how public perceptions about growth had been turned around.

"I think we have a big PR problem here," she said, "starting with a mayor who is obviously prejudiced. Does anyone know more about Melrose? Is there a way to communicate with him?"

"That's a good question," responded Stan Demeral. "We did a little research on the man and he's got quite a history."

"What tragedy was forced on Melrose?" asked Martha Merritt. "It must have been something horrible that makes him so quick to challenge."

"He'd like you to have a vision of him," Stan answered. "A vision of him as tragically handicapped by some accident beyond his control. Actually, Melrose started as a grip-man on a San Francisco Cable Car route. On days off he liked to ride his motorcycle and on one of those days he was involved in an accident that threw him off the vehicle. With the insurance money from the accident he was able to relocate to Minturn."

Stan explained that after winning election to the office of mayor, Melrose decided to become an airplane pilot so that he could more easily connect himself and the town to the outside world. On one of his flights he was forced to make a crash landing and this damaged his lower limbs. Stan granted that Ajax was somewhat biased in saying that he sometimes used his infirmities to encourage approval of his decisions through pity.

"Ajax has to build their team from scratch," Stan continued. "Minturn already has Melrose. His abilities to confront us are not so much in his political expertise as in his persona."

"Rather than confront him, shouldn't we try to meet with him?" asked Martha.

"I think I can arrange that," Peter Newman responded, "Maybe I can get him here before we end this meeting." We took a break for a box lunch sitting on what was once the porch of the mine superintendent. From there you could see that old mine tailings, yellowed by the sulphur brought up with the lead, covered the land down to the river. The breathtaking views across the river were of dark green firs rising up to a tree line at the peak of Mount of the Holy Cross. Some snow still remained in the crossed ravines that gave the peak its name. Newman left the picnic to call Melrose and came back with his report.

"The mayor will see us at two-thirty today. The meeting must be in the Minturn town hall and open to the public. He doesn't want to be accused of doing anything behind closed doors, especially when it comes to Ajax." We all went down to Minturn as requested where a slight man in a wheel chair joined us. This was Melrose. Not James Melrose or Pete Melrose, just Melrose. As the elected mayor, he welcomed us to Minturn as individuals, inferring that some of us might be OK even if we worked for Ajax. Pulling a small notepad from his pocket he read us a quote.

"'*Great things are done when men and mountain meet.*' That ladies and gentlemen is from William Blake's *Gnomic Verses.* I read it to you, because that's my inspiration for living today, to do great things for the town of Minturn." He then

went on to give his idea of greatness: the town wanted to remain as it was. Minturn was already growing because of the expansion of nearby ski resorts and he didn't even want that kind of growth.

The situation was clear. Ajax wanted a mine. Melrose did not. It was easy to admire this man who was able to fight for a cause despite his infirmities. The meeting, of course, ended as soon as it began.

To deal with the opposition, Stan Demeral added more consultants to the team, including experts on economics, grant writing and public relations. Peter Newman said that the first job of the IRC was to develop base-line facts. He wanted statistics on the county economics, social makeup and geography. The task of assessing the environmental impacts of a new mine was assigned to Charlie Gordan. Jella and I were responsible for showing how population growth generated from the mine could be controlled to avoid shantytowns and urban sprawl. Minturn didn't want any of these new folks.

While Jella went to work researching a legal structure that would allow all the planning to take effect, I was given the task of reviewing the Keyser schematic plan. Everyone knew that the present mine buildings were an eyesore. I wanted to put the new buildings underground, but the engineers rejected this idea and balked at a suggestion I made to minimize the mass of the building by rounding off the sharp corner at the roof eaves. I had to hide my prejudices about unimaginative engineers when Ajax asked Keyser Engineers for an estimate of the cost for the idea.

"A million dollars," answered the engineers. I was amazed because the rounded corner is a standard detail for cheap Quonset huts and grain storage bins.

"That's crazy. How about the savings over the typical design?" I asked them later.

"Oh, we didn't calculate that," Keyser replied. "We were only asked to figure the cost."

The team assignments were carried out over a 12 months period in which they established guidelines for controlling every possible impact from the mine. My notes during the first six months showed:

> February 16, 1985: Met Myles Richmond (Town Planner for Minturn) who noted that he feels "his backyard" is being threatened. He guessed that $20 million or more would be speculated to explore the site to see if molybdenum was actually there. That was a drop in the bucket for them. The same amount should be speculated to show Ajax's good faith in doing everything for the

> community they were promising: new schools, a waste treatment plant and the new water system Minturn desperately needs.
>
> February 26, 1985: Trip to Denver to meeting that included new Ajax VP in charge of Gilman mine. He stated his concerns: Short building season, high altitude construction techniques, and low costs.
>
> "All those front end costs for impact reports to answer all those hippies make the project expensive. I wish instead that I was just fighting dinosaurs, but if they were around today we'd be stopped to study them." Everyone smoked: Lucky Strikes!
>
> March 29, 1985: The current attitude in Minturn is "Just make it go away." Their local government has become an adversary rather than a facilitator or policeperson. Its position is to keep the dogs out rather than leash them. A new group will input the countywide socio-economic evaluation. The county was going to be smothered in planning paper.
>
> April 1, 1985: Met Tom, who had moved from Houston, had long hair and a beautiful silver belt buckle that featured carved leaves from a Cannabis bush. He claimed financing for an 850-acre subdivision "just to fill the need". I suspect the project will just be sold as vacation lots to Texans.
>
> June 7, 1985: Met Ralph Cranmore (a man of the city not the hills) and visited the Henderson Mine. Newest hard rock mine in the state. Suited up with hardhat, light and battery, survival kit, belt, boots, safety goggles. Just like putting on ski gear. Elevator dropped us from 10,000 to 5,000 foot level. Operator picks up rock with front-end loader, backs out, dumps on conveyor. Record was +/- 539 passes in one day. That's what it's all about.
>
> June 8, 1985: Meeting of city and county planners. Probably first time they had all talked with each other. I am excited to be in the middle of all this.

My last notes were on June 5, 1986. "Exhaustive feasibility study by economic consultants shows that Gilman project won't fly. Ajax must consider 9 alternative sites." Soon thereafter Ajax told us that rich deposits of Molybdenum had been found in a number of Third World nations. The open market price of the metal fell from $25 to $5 per pound. The Gilman mine was abandoned and the town of Minturn closed back in on itself.

39.

The number of individual suits on the Front Range Casino cases continued to flood Colorado courts while the federal judge made up his mind about the class action suit, but now there was hope for a clear direction from the Federal Court. Despite the fact that individuals had already made settlements at the county and state level, Federal Judge Bright finally decided to certify a mandatory class action suit on the Front Range Casino claims.

During the squabbles about which courts should hear the claims, the Society of Structural Engineers established a panel to investigate the cause of the crash. There would surely be questions from the public as to who was responsible and the Society wanted to be prepared to rebut any claims that the profession produced poor documents or had low ethical standards. Bob Duer was asked to serve on the panel. During its first meeting he showed his slides of the disaster and speculated on possible causes for the failure.

"There were three balconies in the atrium, but levels two and four that stuck out beyond level three failed when they were overloaded. I'll get to the load issues in a minute. The balconies were suspended on one and one half inch diameter rods from the roof framing above. There was no sign of a problem with the size of the roof beams or the connections to the beams. We tested a section of the rod in our lab at CU and found it met the ASTM specifications, in fact was over-designed. The suspension rods were installed as shown in this detail." Bob showed a slide of the connection of the rods at the fourth level beam.

"The initial failure appeared to be where the hanging rods were secured to a box beam at level four. You can see in this slide where the rods were literally

ripped out of the holes at the top of the beam. My first impression was that somehow the box beam had split open."

"So, is that the answer?" asked a member of the panel. "Was the beam just overloaded?" Bob still wasn't sure and adroitly suggested that each panel member take on a different task to examine the problems and that they meet again in three days. When they reassembled, the first member reported as follows:

"I have reviewed all the public records on the construction, including the approved set of working drawings and specifications. The county building department admits that they were never really prepared for such a huge project, and didn't have the expertise to properly check each drawing. There were no provisions in their building code that would have applied to the unusually high occupancy that the casino had that night.

I examined the drawings with that in mind and found that the balconies were only designed for light loads from the few people that would go back and forth to their rooms. Eye witness reports and television pictures taken just before the tragedy show masses of people crowded near the railings of each balcony."

"Who was responsible?" asked one of the panel members.

"The Uniform Building Code used in other parts of the state might have been interpreted by a county inspector to call for much heavier live loads, but the UBC didn't apply in the county. Lacking any local reference, ABC Engineering used a load that was less than 60 percent of that specified in the UBC. Has anyone here studied the connections to see if an overload actually caused the structure to fail?"

"I've had a lot of thoughts about what I saw," answered Bob Duer, "But they are all speculation. Somehow the rod fastening at the box beam gave way and the fourth balcony dropped down on the second balcony and their combined weight crashed to the atrium floor."

When Bob told me about the engineering panel's research, I had an idea about a possible reason for the failure but needed to get more information. Remembering the earlier talk I had with Alberto Gonzalez, I went back to Quebec Avenue and showed him a detail of the rod connections from the original engineering drawings.

"But this is not what we did. The one you have would not be possible to build. Let me show you the drawing that my nephew made. It was submitted and approved by the architects." He produced a 9 by 12 sketch that showed the section where the rods were attached to the fourth floor box beam.

"The engineer wanted to have one continuous rod going through the beam to hold both balcony floors. See on your drawing? Impossible! Impossible to build that way.

We came up with a much better idea. Install one rod going from the ceiling to the fourth floor beam with a nut underneath to hold it. Have another rod to hold up the second floor and attach it to the fourth floor beam by running the rod through it with a nut on the top of the beam."

When Bob Duer saw what Gonzalez had done, he was furious.

"Look at his sketch! See where the two separate rods attach to the forth floor beam. If the original ABC detail had been used, there would have been only one rod and that rod would carry the second floor load all the way to the roof. The Gonzalez drawing shows two shorter rods secured at the top and bottom of the box beam with the same size nut shown on the original engineer's drawing. This put the load of two floors onto a single nut designed to hold only one floor. That nut failed! The devil is in the details."

I reported Bob's findings to Bill Berkowitz who asked me to track down the line of responsibilities and see where someone screwed up. Fernando Gonzales claimed that he had discussed the change with ABC Engineers and they had approved it. ABC didn't agree. Gonzalez should have submitted the drawings to Grabling Construction who would have sent them to Twidley who should have sent them to ABC for review and their stamp that said they conformed to the original shop drawings. Then the stamped drawings should have reversed their flow.

I tried to find out if the paper trail was there. It was, but apparently the papers were just shuffled and never reviewed. No one in the process bothered to look far enough to see the discrepancy between the ABC and Comex drawings. Perhaps the office boys handled everything. If this evidence went to trial, everyone would be found with some degree of fault because each entity had a chance to review the shop drawing. The largest claims would be against ABC because of the live load mistakes found on their drawings plus their lack of attention to the critical connection detail.

Right after Judge Bright authorized a class action suit, some attorneys objected with the claim that Agnes Moore *lacked diversity*, but the federal court finally found four other class representatives. Although this stopped the endless flow of claims by individuals, the class action decision created three different advocacies with differing goals. One represented the plaintiffs, a second the defendants and a third, called *plaintiffs-intervenors*, wanted to disqualify Judge Bright because of communications he'd had with one of the class action representatives.

Although the judge was vindicated of any wrong doing, the class action certification was successfully appealed in Circuit Court: a federal act said that a US court may not stay state court proceedings without authorization from the Con-

gress. The class action proponents then filed various motions to reconsider the appeal, but without success. Nobody seemed to care about the eighty-eight dead and hundreds more injured.

A legal battle evolved between those that wanted to recertify the Federal class action and those who wanted to keep the matter in the state courts. Because both efforts were proceeding in the hopes that they would be successful, Judge Bright finally ordered each side to cooperate with the other. Ultimately the *plaintiffs-intervenors* would join with the defendants to ask for and receive certification of a class action suit in the Tenth District Court. The certification would allow class members to either settle or try for compensatory damages. Finally, all the defendants—owners, casino operators, the county, contractors and subcontractors, engineers and architects—agreed not to contest the liability issue and to establish a $25 million fund for supplemental damages that would be paid in addition to individual compensatory damages awarded by a jury or a mediator. The engineers and architects got a slap on the wrist: their licenses to practice were revoked.

As it was, all the facts I'd uncovered were irrelevant because of the settlement to the class action suit. It was like the answer the judge gave to Sam Lovell's question:

"Justice? Justice? We aren't here to determine justice!"

40.

There was a lull in my work after the settlement on the Front Range Casino; and, I fell into one of those moments of self-doubt that seemed to be endemic with young architects. What was I doing with my life? Yes, I was making good money, but was I really happy doing what I wanted, what I was destined to do? My left-brain was challenging my right brain, and, I guess, my ego was pushing at my id.

Frustration seemed to be a normal condition with architects. Some turned their own lives into one big, continuing architectural problem: taking that jumble of conflicting ideas and trying to turn them into something meaningful. It happened to an old classmate from Utah who had gone on to get a master's degree from Harvard. He and his roommate had equally high grades and graduated from the same venerated Ivy League institution, so what was wrong? His roommate had become the CEO of a start-up electronics company and was making millions while my classmate's wages were lower than a day laborer's.

Classmate decided to seek help and went to a job counselor who put him through a three-day series of vocational tests. Classmate eagerly answered every question, sure that it would lead him into a more rewarding life as a banker or financier. At the completion of the tests, the counselor listed the business and professional opportunities that classmate would be suited for. At the top of the list? Architecture.

I wasn't going to go through the same routine, but I needed to better understand how I fit into a construction world that was becoming more and more complex. Take the Uniform Building Code, the UBC. It was designed to simplify and consolidate rules for making a building safe, but there were hundreds of

new paragraphs added to the Uniform Building Code each time it was revised. To make things worse, every municipality had to adopt the code from a given publication date, and some jurisdictions would adopt the latest edition while others used one from a previous year.

Architecture was becoming more and more intertwined with the law. Actually, it was the other way around. Lawyers were becoming more intertwined with architecture. Lawyers were writing the codes and building laws and then interpreting them. So-called design guidelines were anathemas to creative designers who tried to outsmart them, only to be stopped by a legal interpretation.

Despite the legal implications, architects were marketing themselves as *Master Builders*, capable of designing elaborate structures without a single flaw. One of my favorite magazines warned its readers about their folly with an issue whose cover featured a picture of H. H. Richardson. The turn-of-the century architect was dressed in a hooded monk's robe and it looked as if he'd dribbled food down his full beard. The editorial page described Richardson as a very unconventional individual who nevertheless was respected as a great designer. It went on to point out that the old-time family physician always tried to do his best but never guaranteed results. Then the American Medical Association tried to change the image and turn doctors into infallible gods entrusted with your life. This brought in more patients, but it also brought in the lawyers. The final warning: *Architects Beware.*

Of course, few architects read the editorial and fewer understood where it said they were heading. You couldn't take on a multi-million dollar casino contract and then claim artistic license when the balconies fell down. Each new design twist, each new experiment with materials, each new structural system was supposed to be infallible and it was impossible to blame the almighty when buildings fell apart. A new trend towards architectural stars that were famous for their stylistic shocks didn't help. It was a time when hundred million dollar museums with swoopy-doopy exteriors were filled with leaks and the designer's desktop was covered with lawsuits.

As I reflected on the state of architecture, I was happy with my status. I'd already decided that I couldn't afford to make it as a design dreamer and I could see a fit in my life as a forensic architect. There would be the awful tragedies like Willow Glen or the Front Range Casino. There would be others with simpler solutions like Lodgepole Villas or Cody Place. My recent introduction into the world of environmental impacts gave me a third, and equally intriguing area of work. One thing was sure: there were good guys and bad guys on either side of each case.

The self-appraisal promoted me to clean up the mess in my office that accumulated during the hectic days on Willow Glen and the casino. The floor under

the mail drop was covered with brochures from manufacturers, notices of upcoming AIA meetings, a request to help the Denver Police Association, a Safeway Stores flier announcing this week's sales, bills from the electric and gas companies and one, lone handwritten envelope with a return address in Wolf Creek, Colorado. I separated out the letter, picked up the junk and heaved it in the five-gallon bucket that I used as a wastebasket and carried the bucket out to the dumpster behind the former livery stable.

When I returned, the red light was blinking on my new telephone answering machine. I lost faithful Martha when she decided to become a paralegal and left her switchboard for some brush-up courses at Regis College. The personal touch was lost, but in the long run the machine was a good substitute. Without the human in between, callers were more apt to describe the purpose of their call, giving me a chance to prioritize the order of returning them. There was the usual weekly call from my mother and a message that began and ended with "Dammit." Someone was unhappy to have to talk to the machine. They'd learn. I looked at the letter.

Dear Mr. Stickley:

I have read the newspaper articles about that horrid building collapse up north near Central City. I know it's not for me to say, but I wonder if it wasn't some kind of message from God. Oh, the deaths were dreadful, but maybe they should have never allowed the sinful gambling up there to begin with.

In the newspapers I found your name listed as an architect who was investigating the defects that led to the collapse and obtained your address from the American Institute of Architects. I hope you can help me.

I own a cabin that is part of a new, large ski resort near Wolf Creek. My problem is that I think my house has some construction problems, but the people that built it won't fix them. My neighbors have similar problems.

Please call me if you can help.

Sincerely yours,

Emma Ashforth

Emma had penned a 970 area code number at the bottom of the letter. I thought it was worth a call. She would be in the new resort I'd read about in the

Sunday edition of the *Denver Post.* Stuffed into the massive roll of paper was a full color brochure advertising Wildwood at Wolf Creek. I'd saved a copy and pulled it out of a pile on my desk. The six-page pamphlet gave the history of the new four season recreational resort, with bullets highlighting important features.

- 1000-acre site surrounded by the San Juan National Forest.
- Mesa Resorts, a division of Mesa Timber Corporation.
- Pine forests preserved for your enjoyment.
- Totally planned private community with single-family homes, condominiums and time-share opportunities.
- Eighteen hole golf course designed by famous architect Bobby Whiteside.
- Two lakes and a mountain stream for fly-fishing, kayaking and water sports.
- Ski area for beginners, intermediate and experts: three chairlifts.
- Fritz Kreisel Ski School

A large, colored site plan showed the stream and two lakes, a golf course, clubhouse, ski terrain and base lodge. Separate colors indicated the location of single-family lots, condominiums and a proposed 5 star hotel. The name of architect Neil Beckworth was listed under the rendering of the ski base lodge. I wanted to find out more before calling Emma Ashforth.

Neil said he remembered meeting me, in fact he had seen my name mentioned in regard to that horrible casino disaster. He told me that Colorado architects should rise up against all the carpetbaggers from out of state that didn't understand mountain construction. I knew he was talking about Levey Associates, but didn't want to argue with him about whether they shared any part of the blame.

"So, what brings you to me?" asked Neil. "I hope I don't have any liability problems!"

"No, I saw your name attached to a project called Wildwood at Wolf Creek and hoped you could fill me in on the developer."

"Wow, that's a name out of the past. I did some schematic drawings for a base lodge, but it never went further than that. Just as well, too."

"Were there problems?" Neil paused and then went on to tell me everything he knew about the resort. For starters, he said, the land was originally granted as a mining claim; but, after finding little of interest there, the mining company sold off the acreage to Mesa Timber. Mesa got its start cutting timbers to shore up other mines and they quickly clear-cut everything at the Wolf Creek site.

"What's there now is second growth that's still too small to cut again profitably. What Mesa did was set up a separate corporation called Mesa Resorts. The resort company, with Mesa's backing, borrowed ten million in construction loans from what was then called Watchtower Savings and Loan."

"Ah," I said, "I believe that's the bank controlled by a Mister Hoyt … before he went to jail."

"The story goes that Mesa Resort took three quarters of the construction loan and paid it to Mesa Timber as the supposed purchase price of the property. That put working capital back into the parent firm that was on shaky ground, but left little for Mesa Resort. Publicly, they talked big about prefabrication, using the skills of the parent company, but they could never pre-sell enough of a project to make prefab economical. Prefab needs volume to be effective." Neil told me that they financed the first phase of the project by selling house lots and taking deposits on condominiums. When I told him about her letter, he guessed that Emma would have bought one of those condominiums. He also thought that an in-house architect worked as an employee for Mesa Resorts and designed the condos.

The next day Jella and I made the trip to Wolf Creek. In good weather it was a five-hour drive from Denver, but in winter it took much longer when a blizzard hit Wolf Creek whose annual snowfall of 465 inches was greater than anywhere else in Colorado. We followed Highway 285 that was the most direct route; but the slowest as it made its way through the foothills and down into what was known as South Park, so named by early-day cattlemen who drove their herds north from Texas and grazed them there in the summer months.

Then we passed through Fairplay, another place that claimed to have been visited by gun-slinging Doc Holliday and stopped for lunch at a diner in Alamosa before heading towards Wolf Creek. I almost missed Wildwood. All of a sudden there was a sharp turn to the left as the road reached the edge of a ridge and turned to start down across the contours. The panorama of Wolf Creek Valley spread out below. As we slowed to take in the view, I realized that we'd gone too far and turned around where the road widened at the hairpin turn.

A quarter mile further back on the left I saw a side road that had been obscured by trees on our first pass. A ranch gate made of varnished logs carried a

sign for Wildwood. On each side of the road, small signs called out the lot numbers. We stopped at a gatehouse whose occupant was eager to sell us property. When I asked the directions to Emma Ashforth's, the guard/salesperson urged us to come inside where she could identify Emma's unit on their scale model. She wasn't about to lose potential customers.

Jella and I looked at a site replica that was at least twelve feet square. The green painted Styrofoam was shaped to show the ski hill, the creek and the lakes. Hundreds of small wood squares grouped along the golf course indicated houses. Larger blocks carried ubiquitous resort names for condos, the hotel and the ski lodge. The salesperson showed us an area called The Pines and the road to follow to find Emma's condominium.

Back in the car, it wasn't long before we found a cluster of units that were all separated from each other like tourist cabins in a national park. Emma's was the only unit in sight with a car parked in front. The other owners were not at home or were non-existent: ghosts in another see-through project without shades or curtains to indicate occupancy.

Emma Ashforth greeted us in a green ranger's shirt, matching pants, a Forest Service name badge and Gore-Tex walking shoes. I guessed she was in her middle fifties. Her graying hair was cut short suggesting a lot of time spent outdoors. When she invited us in, I quickly guessed that she was single, and lived alone except for the big, black Newfoundland stretched out before a darkened fireplace. The dog stretched, turned towards us and started to get up.

"Don't worry about Fritz," she said. "He's just a big teddy bear and loves to be patted. You are so nice to come all the way down here with … what's your name again, dear? Oh yes, Angela. And you are an attorney you say? Maybe we need you too." Emma suggested that before we sat down we look at her front porch. Outside, I could see that four, six-by-six posts held up her porch roof. She pointed near the floor.

"See where all the posts sit on those concrete piers? You can see some that look like they are rotting already and this place is hardly five years old. Now over here look at the walls of this cabin. See how they have been pushed in, pushed out of shape?" She reached down to scratch Fritz behind the ears. "Let's go have some coffee."

While Emma moved around her small kitchen she told us about herself. She was an employee of the US Forest Service. She and her husband Dave had lived in Alamosa for twenty-five years until an avalanche tragically wiped him out when they were making a backcountry tour. She took her small inheritance and

bought in Wildwood. She liked the location and assumed that her investment was safe and would improve in value as the resort was built out.

"This was to be the first-ever, year-round mountain resort built from scratch. As a ranger, I've known and worked for years with people from Mesa Timber. They of course were out for profit but they always abided by USFS rules. The promoters of the resort are different, you know, from Mesa Timber even though they have the same name. Before Dave went, we'd go to parties where busloads of would-be customers unloaded from as far away as Tucson. The promoters were all just handshaking salespeople that came here from Arizona and California and as far away as Hawaii."

"I've met some of those super-sales people. They just trade their suede shoes for cowboy boots and keep on talking the same talk." I hoped I hadn't hit on some of her friends.

"Well, it's taken me a while to learn, but you're right. The salespeople blew in here like humming birds when the project first opened and then flew away when things slowed down. Up until the real estate crash, they were flying prospects into a new strip they'd built in Pagosa Springs. 'Made it big enough to bring in 757's. Now it's all just weeds."

Jella and I left Emma to walk again around the twenty-odd buildings actually built of the one hundred proposed for The Pines. I mentioned my surprise that the project was called a condominium, but that all the units were detached. Jella explained that the legal form gave the developers a platform to control the architectural designs. It also created an association that was empowered to charge fees for the maintenance of the common grounds. This assured Mesa that their first project would be a showcase for future sales. I had another thought.

"Jella, look at these units. If you squint your eyes, they could be large mobile homes. I'll bet that Mesa planned to mass-produce these units in a remote plant and drag them to the site. They never pre-sold enough to make it profitable to pre-fab these, but they built some models here as if they were trailers."

We stopped at one of the units where the walls had begun to cave in. I looked through a crack and could see that the walls were made up of two-by-fours with plywood attached inside and out. This created a sandwich panel similar to the walls used on house and truck trailers; but it hardly met local codes that required two-by-six studs that were deep enough to hold the thick insulation needed in snow country.

Dark stains left by heavy snowfalls girded the lower sidewalls of the unit. I looked up at the metal roof and could see that it was steep enough to shed even the lightest snowfall. I had a theory.

"These roofs were designed to shed snow A.S.A.P in order to avoid loading the roof rafters. This allowed them to use much smaller timbers than normally found around here. When all 465 inches that came off the roofs piled up against the sidewalls, the pressure from the snow would have buckled those lightweight walls. It would have been like holding a chunk of cheese in your hand and then squeezing it tightly. Squish, squish, and boom! The sides collapse."

"What about the dry rot at the posts?" Jella asked.

"The wood was sitting directly on those concrete piers, so moisture that settled on the piers was sucked up by the posts. In ski areas up north, there wouldn't be a problem; but down here the moisture content is so high that it's like being in California where they isolate any wood from potentially damaging water."

"Here we go again, Woody. It's a bona fide class action problem. We probably would get nothing for Emma and the others from the resort company; but we can prove that, as a subsidiary, it's a creature of the parent corporation and go after Mesa Timber. They are going to have to replace all of these units with properly designed ones. It's no fun seeing all this after the fact. There'd be no problem if they'd done it right in the first place."

41.

It was late in the afternoon by the time we completed the paperwork with Emma. Jella assured her that she'd be compensated for every penny she'd invested in The Pines and a fair amount for the hardships imposed on her by Mesa Resorts. She also advised her to be looking around for a more secure real estate investment as soon as she received the settlement money. We needed a list of all the other owners and Emma assured us that she could get it because of her friendship with the gatekeeper.

"After all," she said, "in a small town like this we band together because we're all in the same boat. In this case, Mesa Timber owns the boat."

Jella would pick up the case from there, first contacting the half dozen other people that had purchased a unit to include them as participants in her threat to a class action suit. She would then notify Mesa Timber that they'd better compensate all the buyers or face litigation. I would document the structural defects that would back up her claim. As we drove away from The Pines, I had an idea.

"Jella, I understand that there's an historic hotel down the road in Durango; and I'd like to take a look at it. Why don't we spend the night down here?"

"It depends upon how much of this will be research and how much will be ..."

"I believe in combining, wherever it's possible to conserve energy."

"Hopefully, you won't try to conserve too much of it." So, we headed down the steep grade into Wolf Creek Valley, through Pagosa Springs and then on to Durango. We talked again about how different the San Juan Mountains seemed from those up north. The heavier rainfall brought out a lush evergreen growth in

contrast to the spindly lodgepole pines in Summit County. The road followed along the San Juan River and soon became the main street in Durango.

"Look at that." Jella pointed to the tallest building in town, a four-story structure with a three-story wing. The red brick walls were accented by a grab bag collection of white painted arches, cornices and buttresses at the building corners to hold up an overscaled projecting parapet. This was the Hotel Strater.

While I signed us in, Jella was taking brochures from a rack in the hotel lobby. After getting the pass key, we walked up three stories, entered a room filled with Victorian furniture and Jella sat down on the four-poster bed to read me the brochure highlights.

"This was built in 1887 by a young pharmacist named Henry Strater. Henry wanted the big building to highlight a drug store that he planned to put on the street level. More interested in pharmaceuticals than running a hotel, he leased the building to H. L. Rice. Unfortunately, he neglected to separate the drug store space from the lease and Rice turned around and charged him an exorbitant rent."

"Enough!" I interrupted, "Let's go have a drink."

"There's just a little more," She pleaded. "The Strater Hotel contains 376,000 red bricks that were made locally, employing the same techniques used here by Native Americans many centuries before."

"Native Americans made bricks here centuries ago?" I asked. As Jella opened another brochure, I moved towards her in the hope that a kiss would end the dissertation. I wasn't fast enough.

"This area was the center of an Anasazi culture that thrived here from 600 to 1300. Just a little west of here is Mesa Verde and the mis-named town of Aztec. It says here that the closest Aztecs were 1500 miles away to the south, but the early settlers used the only word they knew to describe the ancient tribes." I thought about holding my hand over her mouth instead of kissing her, and then I realized she was just trying to get a rise out of me and I didn't want to be her victim. I'd learned a lot about holding my temper since the days of having my hat thrown into a tree. I took a deep breath and tried to sound nonchalant.

"A plan. Let's have a drink downstairs in the saloon, find a place to eat and get to bed early. Tomorrow morning we can drive down to Aztec and then over to Mesa Verde before we go home.

In Aztec, we found a number of 700-year-old ruins made out of bricks like the ones duplicated on the Strater Hotel. The most impressive sight was the wall that remained of a huge, circular Kiva or assembly area for tribal events. We were looking at the remains of a civilization that was as old as the Anglo-Saxons that

invaded England. This all gave me a new slant about American History. It didn't start with the Pilgrims. Here was evidence of the real Americans that somehow disappeared in 1300. No one knows why. They had to be very advanced to have built all of the structures whose remains lay before us. I was proud of these people and pleased to be standing in what was literally the birthplace of an American culture. Albeit lost to us now, it all started here.

Aztec was just a warm-up for Mesa Verde, where the Anasazi built hundreds of elaborate homes and public structures under huge rock overhangs. The ranger took our fee at the entrance to the National Park and handed us an information sheet that described the many unanswered questions surrounding the site. Why did the same tribe that created the Aztec ruins decide to build such an inaccessible place? Was it for religious purposes or for their defense? What happened in the 14th Century that made them vacate the village? The answers weren't apparent when we checked out the Cliff House structures high above the parking lot. To get there, we climbed a set of ladders and only found scant remains of some of the 150 rooms and little evidence as to how or why they were actually occupied.

On our return to Denver we went back through Durango and headed north on the steep grade up through Silverton to Ouray. As we hit Red Mountain Pass we were side-by-side with a steam locomotive carrying tourists on the railroad tracks that served the old silver mines. On each side of the road we could see tailings and old mine shafts. We paused at a sign commemorating the National Belle mine that told how the miners broke through a layer of rock to find natural caves with silver literally hanging from the ceilings.

We stopped for lunch in Ouray and sat at a table in the restaurant's small garden. Pots of bright red geraniums accented a wall. I was enervated both by what we'd learned on our morning tours and the beauty of the mountains around us. It seemed like a good time to share my thoughts about things that would make a major change in my life.

"This has been a great trip. As you know, I've never been out of the Rocky Mountains and have never visited the historic cities of Europe; but here we've seen evidence of hundreds of years of our own American history. I'm beginning to see that architecture, and the Aztecs certainly invented our earliest architecture, was and is something more than just a series of styles. It's a fabric woven from the multiple histories of each culture.

"That's where I see Woody Stickley fitting in. I want to build a practice that worries about that fabric. It will all unravel if we don't find ways to stop depleting our non-renewable natural resources. With Ajax we had a chance to influence where and how a building could be built with sustainable materials and conserve

energy. Think of how much it takes to resurrect a construction failure. I don't expect to be put on the cover of *Time* for my work, but this gives me a direction I can believe in.

"This means I'll need to make some changes. Because of you, I am sort of a recognized expert in investigating building failures. The more their reasons can be discovered, the more we can eliminate them. I've also got a foot in the door as a consultant on environmental impacts. It's time to build on that and I'd like to expand the office. Perhaps I can get Bob Duer to become a partner and there should be enough business to support a small office staff. The biggest question I have is whether to include a legal partner. There's no question about who that would be, but I'm not sure that's the best way to proceed."

"Woody! I've been hoping this would happen. I've thought often about starting just such a business with you; but, like you, I'm not sure that's the best way to go. I think I can do more through Bates Brown & Berkowitz and I also think it might be best for our … our relationship."

I dropped Jella off at her house and drove over to Larimer Square to catch up on office work that had been put off by our trip south.

42.

One of the calls on my answering machine was from Sam Lovell at Smith & Bair Architects. He said their firm had a problem with a swimming pool addition to a hotel in Boulder. Could I meet him tomorrow at the site?

I drove down 28th Street in Boulder until I saw a sign for the Hearthstone. Under the hotel name was the phrase *A Luxury Lodging Hotel* and under that an AAA logo. Sam had a roll of drawings under his arm when we met at the parking lot. He told me that the hotel had changed hands a number of times during the past ten years, but had been recently purchased by a local group who saved the name but changed the franchise to the Luxury Lodging chain. We walked into the lobby and then turned left into the newly completed addition that was designed by Smith & Bair. Just inside the new wing, a long wall of glass separated the corridor from a room with tiled walls and floors and a small swimming pool.

Sam led me to the edge of the pool and pointed towards a bright chromium handrail that led down some steps into the pool. I could see that it sloped with the steps and ended under water.

"A month ago," said Sam," a guest of the hotel came in here and, possibly after a few drinks, dove into the pool. Unfortunately, he failed to read the warning signs that prohibited diving and landed on the part of the railing that is under water. Yesterday, we received a notice from New Jersey that named Smith & Bair, the general contractor, the pool contractor and Luxury Lodging as defendants in a suit filed in Newark on behalf of Clint Rodham. According to the suit, Clint was in great pain from a broken shoulder and various other contusions received when he dove into the Hearthstone pool. He's suing for the cost of a

Medvac flight to his hospital in Teaneck, medical expenses and an amount of $100,000 for pain and suffering."

Sam unrolled the drawings that showed how they indicated the outline of a pool, but stated in bold type that a separate pool contractor was responsible for its design and construction. There was no indication of steps into the pool or a handrail on the Smith & Bair drawings. Sam said that a judge had insisted on a pre-trial meeting of all parties that was scheduled for the following Wednesday. Unfortunately, Sam had a deadline to complete construction documents for a major high-rise on that day.

"Would you and that nice lady lawyer take this off my hands?" he asked. "We have no responsibility here, but you know how they do this. 'Name everybody and hope that one of us is guilty."

Jella said that she could take on the suit, providing that it could be cleaned up quickly because she had a trial starting on the following week. While she looked up New Jersey law, I went into the Boulder building department and looked over all the drawings that they had on the project. Yes, the architects' drawings left the pool's design and construction up to a pool contractor. I found that Bright Pools was awarded the contract, but their drawings didn't show any handrail either. I was baffled and asked to see the building inspector who had checked the work in progress. He had no answer to my question about who was responsible for the handrail, but then remembered something about the job.

"Yeah, the pool was in and we were going to give the whole job a certificate of occupancy, but at the last minute the board of health guy said that he wouldn't sign off. He insisted that the railing be installed and that according to code it had to extend eighteen inches beyond the top and bottom steps. Of course when you are waist deep in water on the bottom step you don't need a handrail, but he stuck to the code."

We got an early morning flight to Newark and arrived in time for the meeting. Jella didn't say much on the flight, but spent the time looking over notes she had on New Jersey law. At the meeting place we found the judge, a court recorder, representatives for the general contractor, their liability insurance carrier and the attorneys for their insurance company. Similar trios were present for Bright Pools and Luxury Lodging.

The attorney representing Clint Rodham said that his client was still bedridden and unable to attend the conference. He started the proceedings by citing the numerous injuries caused by the defendants. He admitted that Clint had had a social highball with a friend before he entered the pool area, but claimed that Clint never saw any signs prohibiting diving. They were on the back of the

entrance door. There was no way that Clint would have seen them unless he'd turned around.

The attorney for the general contractor commented that the pool was small and obviously not a diving pool and wondered how Mr. Rodham could even think it was a diving pool unless he, perhaps, had more to drink than he'd admitted. The attorney further claimed that the general contractor was only following the drawings given to him and that the fault lay elsewhere.

Jella picked up on the statement and asked me to show the drawings prepared by the architect. She insisted that her client bore no guilt and didn't deserve such harassment. Then, she looked at her notes and spoke to the group.

"I don't know why this suit was filed in New Jersey, but it was. Under New Jersey law, a suit may not be brought against any party unless that party lives or does business within the state." Glances were exchanged around the room and some began to put away their papers and close briefcases. The general contractor group and the Luxury Lodging group rose in unison. The Bright Pool people sat still, knowing that they were licensed to build pools in all 50 states. The judge smiled and nodded agreement that the rest were free to leave.

I smiled at Jella and shook my head in wonderment.

"I don't know what we architects would do without you lawyers. What a deal!"

"We should celebrate."

"First, I was hoping that you might like to see where all the Stickley roots were planted. It's not far from here to Parsippany-Troy Hills."

"Person penny where?' She laughed as we got into the rental car I'd driven from the airport.

43.

We drove the thirty miles along I-280 to Parsippany-Troy Hills. When we arrived there I began to wonder if something might have happened to the family homestead. Since our visit from Salt Lake City many years before, the town seemed to have been swamped by industry. According to the Chamber of Commerce sign at the edge of town, it was host to 53 of the *Fortune 500* companies. Just beyond that sign we happily found an official white-on-green one with a directional arrow for Craftsman Farms.

It wasn't hard to find. One sign at the entrance announced it as a National Historic Landmark. Gustav would have liked that. Another sign said that it was an Official Project of Save America's Treasures. Gustav would have liked that also. When I mentioned Gustav's name to Jella, I realized there were some things I'd better tell her about my ancestor.

"His furniture was and still is beautifully simple and yet elegant. The furniture fitted his theory about *a fine plainness* in the arts, but Gustav also wanted to apply it to what he called the art of living. As soon as he made some money he jumped into social philosophy with a vengeance. He needed a venue to display his unconventional ideas and moved his home from Syracuse, New York to what was then rural property in this town. He bought up dozens of individual parcels that added up to more than six hundred acres.

"Gustav wanted all that acreage to create his ideal community. There would be a farm school for boys. Vegetables from the farm gardens and fruit from the orchards plus dairy cows and chickens would allow his colony to become self-sufficient. His first move in his *Garden of Eden* was to construct the Club House that

was meant to be a gathering place for students, workers and guests attracted to his philosophy."

"Sounds just like a Stickley to me," Jella chided. "So what happened to the Garden of Eden?"

"The Club house was set up with a kitchen and meeting room to serve over one hundred people but it was never put to use. When the Craftsman style lost popularity, furniture sales dropped. Gustav wasn't able to build a separate house for his wife and four daughters, so they all moved into the second floor of the Club House until around 1915."

"What happened then?"

"Then he went into bankruptcy and lost the property. Not a good omen for the rest of the Stickleys."

As we drove up the driveway it was easy to pick out the Club House that was made out of hand-hewn logs and local stone. Inside, we walked first into the dining room. On one of the log walls a sideboard that must have been ten feet long had the simple grace that Gustav was known for. Wrought iron hinges spread across what looked like quartered oak doors. Rails above the countertop held wine goblets and platters. A card on the counter described the piece as an authentic reproduction from a design that first appeared on the cover of *American Cabinet Maker.*

Other furniture in the room included glass-front corner cabinets. A reproduction of a 1906 *Craftsman* magazine showed similar cabinets under a text that warned:

> *This piece is the most difficult of any yet given in our Cabinet Work series. The glass mullions ... demanded careful work.*

This kind of complicated detail for a supposedly simple piece reminded me of furniture that modern designers were pushing in the late 1950's. The idea then was to make supposedly cheap chairs out of plain metal rods and bent plywood. In order to get something the average person could sit in, the plywood had to be molded with curves and the rods secured with complicated fasteners. The resulting pieces cost more than the chairs from Grand Rapids that they were mass-producing with intricately turned legs and brass-nailed leather seats.

In the great hall or living room, we were impressed by a unique Stickley upright piano. For one who only knew the name Steinway, this was a surprise. The light oak panels were inlaid with pewter and tinted woods that pictured styl-

ized plant stems and bright blossoms. After looking at other pieces, particularly ones that we agreed we'd like to have in our home, we could see how Gustav's appetite was larger than his pocketbook. If he'd had the money, would his social idea have been tested at his Garden of Eden? Would his commune have saved its residents money? As in today's world, did they have to spend half of the cost of anything getting it from the point of production to our homes?

Gustav's Garden of Eden would have nicely answered a growing need that environmentalists were voicing to reduce energy costs, minimize the use of non-renewable resources and produce organic foods. He, along with other Utopians, was asking for changes in the fabric of a civilization that he could hardly have anticipated and would never see. I'd have to change my mind about my ancestor's ideas about the art of living.

Jella picked up a few brochures about Craftsman Farms as we walked out the door of the Club House. Driving back to the Newark Airport, I suddenly felt the rental car begin to shake and realized that we had a tire problem. I pulled off the highway onto the shoulder and looked in the trunk for a spare that was not there. Now what? We waited for some kind of help to come along, expecting the New Jersey state Highway Patrol to be all over the place to collect speeding fines. Ten minutes. Twenty minutes. They probably were all in Atlantic City pretending to look for criminals that they'd never find. As we sat there, I thought about Gustav, but mostly about something else. Jella finally broke the silence.

"What's on your mind, architect?" I was slow to respond.

"That's a second thing that I wanted to talk to you about. Actually it's more important but harder to express than my thoughts in Ouray. I know it's getting shopworn, but the analogy about fabric doesn't end with architecture. I feel that at last I'm coming to know myself. Lot's of those loose threads have been untangled and made into whole cloth.

"We talked earlier about the two of us starting a service organization. In addition to your being in a better position by staying with BB&B, I don't think we should do anything that might affect what you call our professional relationship. That one degree of separation may be best for our professional lives, but I have other ideas about the rest of the time." I rested my left arm on the wheel and carefully phrased my next statement.

"Jella, will you marry me?" Her hazel eyes focused on mine. If she'd been looking for some sign of hesitation or doubt, my own eyes gave her an answer. She didn't quickly answer my question, but placed both of her hands over my free right hand and slowly shook her head; but I wasn't sure which way.

Just then I turned to see who was rapping on the car window. It was a highway patrolman who had stopped to see if we needed help. After my explaining our predicament he radioed for a tow truck. We were dragged to a nearby garage and the mechanic removed an ancient square nail from the tire: our gift from Gustav Stickley. When the tire was replaced and we got back into the car, Jella looked at me and said,

"Just drive right by the airport. Head for the tunnel and New York City. We're going to spend the night at the St. Regis on the Smith and Bair account. Tomorrow we'll walk up and down Fifth Avenue. I'll be shopping for a wedding dress.

978-0-595-46819-5
0-595-46819-5

Printed in the United States
112768LV00003B/244/P

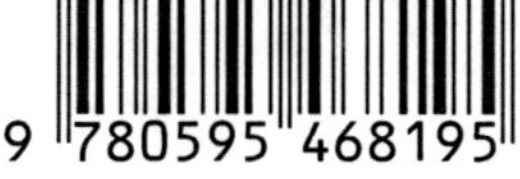

THE TOTAL TORSO PROGRAM

Program Component	Mon /	Tues /	Wed /	Thur /	Fri /	Sat /	Sun /
Knees to Chest							
Modified Plow							
Torso Twist							
Back Machine							
Back Extensions							
Extensions Off Table							
Abdominal Machine							
Curl-Ups							
Leg Throws							
Assisted Leg Throws							
Leg Exchange							
Leg Exchange with Twist							
Aerobic Work (Type, duration, intensity, misc.)							

Under *day of week:* Insert date at slash (e.g., 10/31).
For *Machines:* Note intensity setting and number of reps.
For *Stretching:* Note time held and repetitions.
For *Calisthenics:* Note number of repetitions.
For *Aerobics:* Note data as listed in left-hand column.

THE TOTAL TORSO PROGRAM

Program Component	Mon /	Tues /	Wed /	Thur /	Fri /	Sat /	Sun /
Knees to Chest							
Modified Plow							
Torso Twist							
Back Machine							
Back Extensions							
Extensions Off Table							
Abdominal Machine							
Curl-Ups							
Leg Throws							
Assisted Leg Throws							
Leg Exchange							
Leg Exchange with Twist							
Aerobic Work (Type, duration, intensity, misc.)							

Under *day of week:* Insert date at slash (e.g., 10/31).
For *Machines:* Note intensity setting and number of reps.
For *Stretching:* Note time held and repetitions.
For *Calisthenics:* Note number of repetitions.
For *Aerobics:* Note data as listed in left-hand column.

THE TOTAL TORSO PROGRAM

Program Component	Mon /	Tues /	Wed /	Thur /	Fri /	Sat /	Sun /
Knees to Chest							
Modified Plow							
Torso Twist							
Back Machine							
Back Extensions							
Extensions Off Table							
Abdominal Machine							
Curl-Ups							
Leg Throws							
Assisted Leg Throws							
Leg Exchange							
Leg Exchange with Twist							
Aerobic Work (Type, duration, intensity, misc.)							

Under *day of week:* Insert date at slash (e.g., 10/31).
For *Machines:* Note intensity setting and number of reps.
For *Stretching:* Note time held and repetitions.
For *Calisthenics:* Note number of repetitions.
For *Aerobics:* Note data as listed in left-hand column.

THE TOTAL TORSO PROGRAM

Program Component	Mon /	Tues /	Wed /	Thur /	Fri /	Sat /	Sun /
Knees to Chest							
Modified Plow							
Torso Twist							
Back Machine							
Back Extensions							
Extensions Off Table							
Abdominal Machine							
Curl-Ups							
Leg Throws							
Assisted Leg Throws							
Leg Exchange							
Leg Exchange with Twist							
Aerobic Work (Type, duration, intensity, misc.)							

Under *day of week:* Insert date at slash (e.g., 10/31).
For *Machines:* Note intensity setting and number of reps.
For *Stretching:* Note time held and repetitions.
For *Calisthenics:* Note number of repetitions.
For *Aerobics:* Note data as listed in left-hand column.

THE TOTAL TORSO PROGRAM

Program Component	Mon /	Tues /	Wed /	Thur /	Fri /	Sat /	Sun /
Knees to Chest							
Modified Plow							
Torso Twist							
Back Machine							
Back Extensions							
Extensions Off Table							
Abdominal Machine							
Curl-Ups							
Leg Throws							
Assisted Leg Throws							
Leg Exchange							
Leg Exchange with Twist							
Aerobic Work (Type, duration, intensity, misc.)							

Under *day of week:* Insert date at slash (e.g., 10/31).
For *Machines:* Note intensity setting and number of reps.
For *Stretching:* Note time held and repetitions.
For *Calisthenics:* Note number of repetitions.
For *Aerobics:* Note data as listed in left-hand column.

THE TOTAL TORSO PROGRAM

Program Component	Mon /	Tues /	Wed /	Thur /	Fri /	Sat /	Sun /
Knees to Chest							
Modified Plow							
Torso Twist							
Back Machine							
Back Extensions							
Extensions Off Table							
Abdominal Machine							
Curl-Ups							
Leg Throws							
Assisted Leg Throws							
Leg Exchange							
Leg Exchange with Twist							
Aerobic Work (Type, duration, intensity, misc.)							

Under *day of week:* Insert date at slash (e.g., 10/31).
For *Machines:* Note intensity setting and number of reps.
For *Stretching:* Note time held and repetitions.
For *Calisthenics:* Note number of repetitions.
For *Aerobics:* Note data as listed in left-hand column.

THE TOTAL TORSO PROGRAM

Program Component	Mon /	Tues /	Wed /	Thur /	Fri /	Sat /	Sun /
Knees to Chest							
Modified Plow							
Torso Twist							
Back Machine							
Back Extensions							
Extensions Off Table							
Abdominal Machine							
Curl-Ups							
Leg Throws							
Assisted Leg Throws							
Leg Exchange							
Leg Exchange with Twist							
Aerobic Work (Type, duration, intensity, misc.)							

Under *day of week:* Insert date at slash (e.g., 10/31).
For *Machines:* Note intensity setting and number of reps.
For *Stretching:* Note time held and repetitions.
For *Calisthenics:* Note number of repetitions.
For *Aerobics:* Note data as listed in left-hand column.

THE TOTAL TORSO PROGRAM

Program Component	Mon /	Tues /	Wed /	Thur /	Fri /	Sat /	Sun /
Knees to Chest							
Modified Plow							
Torso Twist							
Back Machine							
Back Extensions							
Extensions Off Table							
Abdominal Machine							
Curl-Ups							
Leg Throws							
Assisted Leg Throws							
Leg Exchange							
Leg Exchange with Twist							
Aerobic Work (Type, duration, intensity, misc.)							

Under *day of week:* Insert date at slash (e.g., 10/31).
For *Machines:* Note intensity setting and number of reps.
For *Stretching:* Note time held and repetitions.
For *Calisthenics:* Note number of repetitions.
For *Aerobics:* Note data as listed in left-hand column.

THE TOTAL TORSO PROGRAM

Program Component	Mon /	Tues /	Wed /	Thur /	Fri /	Sat /	Sun /
Knees to Chest							
Modified Plow							
Torso Twist							
Back Machine							
Back Extensions							
Extensions Off Table							
Abdominal Machine							
Curl-Ups							
Leg Throws							
Assisted Leg Throws							
Leg Exchange							
Leg Exchange with Twist							
Aerobic Work (Type, duration, intensity, misc.)							

Under *day of week:* Insert date at slash (e.g., 10/31).
For *Machines:* Note intensity setting and number of reps.
For *Stretching:* Note time held and repetitions.
For *Calisthenics:* Note number of repetitions.
For *Aerobics:* Note data as listed in left-hand column.

THE TOTAL TORSO PROGRAM

Program Component	Mon /	Tues /	Wed /	Thur /	Fri /	Sat /	Sun /
Knees to Chest							
Modified Plow							
Torso Twist							
Back Machine							
Back Extensions							
Extensions Off Table							
Abdominal Machine							
Curl-Ups							
Leg Throws							
Assisted Leg Throws							
Leg Exchange							
Leg Exchange with Twist							
Aerobic Work (Type, duration, intensity, misc.)							

Under *day of week:* Insert date at slash (e.g., 10/31).
For *Machines:* Note intensity setting and number of reps.
For *Stretching:* Note time held and repetitions.
For *Calisthenics:* Note number of repetitions.
For *Aerobics:* Note data as listed in left-hand column.